D1515355

Advanced
EXERCISES IN DIAGNOSTIC RADIOLOGY

11

THE CERVICAL SPINE IN TRAUMA

AMIL J. GERLOCK, Jr., M.D.
Associate Professor of Radiology, Chief of Angiography

SANDRA G. KIRCHNER, M.D.
Assistant Professor of Radiology, Director of Medical Student Education

RICHARD M. HELLER, M.D.
Associate Professor of Radiology, Director of Pediatric Radiology

JEREMY J. KAYE, M.D.
Associate Professor of Radiology, Chief—Section of Bone and Joint Radiology

All of Vanderbilt University Hospital, Department of Radiology and Radiologic Sciences, Nashville, Tennessee

W. B. SAUNDERS COMPANY • PHILADELPHIA • LONDON • TORONTO

W. B. Saunders Company: West Washington Square
                         Philadelphia, PA 19105

                         1 St. Anne's Road
                         Eastbourne, East Sussex BN21 3UN, England

                         1 Goldthorne Avenue
                         Toronto, Ontario M8Z 5T9, Canada

Library of Congress Cataloging in Publication Data
Main entry under title:

The Cervical spine in trauma.

    (Advanced exercises in diagnostic radiology; 11)
    1. Vertebrae, Cervical—Wounds and injuries—Diagnosis. 2. Vertebrae,
Cervical—Radiography.
I. Gerlock, Amil J.
RC78.E89 vol. 11 [RD633] 616.07′57s [617′.1] 77-16983
ISBN 0-7216-4115-6

Advanced Exercises in Diagnostic Radiology—11

THE CERVICAL SPINE IN TRAUMA   ISBN 0-7216-4115-6

Last digit is the print number: 9   8   7   6   5

PREFACE

Except to control hemorrhage and establish a patent airway, you must not move the head and neck of patients who have sustained trauma to the neck until you have studied a lateral radiograph of the cervical spine. There are few moments in medicine when the correct on-the-spot radiologic interpretation is more crucial to the management of a patient than the moment when you view this initial lateral radiograph of the cervical spine of an acutely injured patient. The lateral view is the only projection that can be readily obtained without moving the patient's head and neck. From this view alone, you must make the initial determination of fracture or no fracture, subluxation or no subluxation, and normal or abnormal. Thus, the emphasis in this text is on the lateral roentgenogram.

This monograph is written for you, the physician evaluating the cervical spine of an acutely injured patient.

It should be stressed that this text does not cover all of the possible traumatic abnormalities of the cervical spine but emphasizes the approach.

ACKNOWLEDGMENTS

The authors express their deep gratitude to Ms. Dorthy Gutekunst and Mr. John Bobbitt for their photography and to Ms. Kayan Rogers for assistance in the preparation of the manuscript. The authors also wish to thank Dr. William Hunter for reviewing the manuscript and Dr. A. Everette James, Jr., for his encouragement.

CONTENTS

CONTENTS

INTRODUCTION

This monograph is intended to serve as a basic guide to the interpretation of radiographs of the cervical spine in trauma. You can obtain optimal benefit from this text by first reviewing the sections on normal anatomy. The remainder of the roentgenograms of the cervical spine should then be looked upon as unknowns. Space is provided after each unknown radiograph for you to record your answers to the following four questions:

1. Which anatomic structure or structures are involved?
2. Are the involved structures displaced or nondisplaced?
3. Is this a stable or an unstable injury?
4. What is the common eponym or diagnostic term for the type of injury seen on the radiograph?

Question three deserves special comment. While it is our intention to deal primarily with correct roentgen diagnosis, the determination of stability is important because this condition governs immediate patient management, including whether to obtain additional roentgenographic views and even whether to move the patient to a radiographic table.

The question of stability is, however, a difficult one, over which there is often considerable controversy. For our purposes, a fracture is considered stable if the patient may be safely moved with caution without the risk of additional injury.

After you have recorded your answers, turn the page and study the answer sheet and the line drawings provided.

A short discussion is found in each chapter.

The final test cases, in Chapter 17, differ in that the questions are multiple choice. Any or all choices may be correct. The answers to the questions are found at the end of the chapter.

CHAPTER 1

NORMAL RADIOGRAPHIC ANATOMY OF THE LATERAL VIEW OF THE CERVICAL SPINE

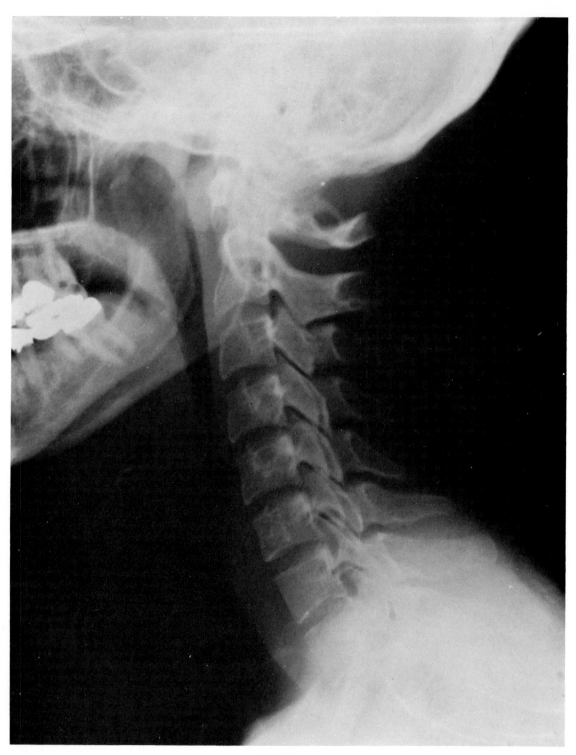

FIGURE 1

Can you identify each of the anatomic structures listed below on the lateral radiograph of the cervical spine on the opposite page?

1. Occipital condyle of the skull

2. Posterior margin of the foramen magnum

3. Odontoid process or dens of C-2

4. Anterior arch of C-1

5. Posterior arch of C-1

6. C-2 vertebral body

7. Space between the posterior surface of the anterior arch of C-1 and anterior surface of the odontoid process

8. Pedicle of C-6

9. Superior articular process of C-4

10. Inferior articular process of C-5

11. Intervertebral disc space between C-5 and C-6

12. Tip of the spinous process of C-7

13. Lamina of C-3

14. Base of the spinous process of C-3

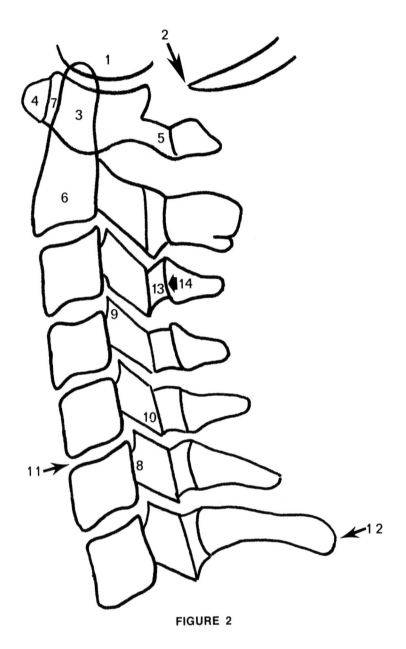

FIGURE 2

Name the anatomic structures numbered on the diagram (Fig. 2) of the lateral radiograph of the cervical spine.

1. _____

2. _____

3. _____

4. _____

5. _____

6. _____

7. _____

8. _____

9. _____

10. _____

11. _____

12. _____

13. _____

14. _____

You have already seen the answers, of course; they are listed on the previous page.

CHAPTER 2

THE FOUR CONTOUR LINES OF THE CERVICAL SPINE: NORMAL ANATOMY

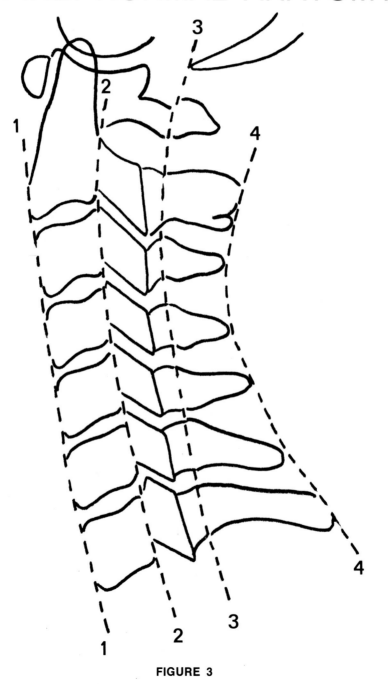

FIGURE 3

Four Contour Lines of the
Cervical Spine

The four contour lines of the cervical spine are illustrated in Figure 3.

1. A smooth gentle curve, convex anteriorly, should be formed by a line drawn along the anterior margins of the cervical vertebral bodies (dotted line 1).

2. A smooth gentle curve, convex anteriorly, should be formed by a line drawn along the posterior margins of the cervical vertebral bodies (dotted line 2). This outlines the anterior margin of the spinal canal.

3. A smooth gentle curve, convex anteriorly, should be formed by a line drawn along the anterior margins of the bases of the spinous processes (dotted line 3). This outlines the posterior margin of the spinal canal and is called the *spinolaminal line.*

4. A smooth gentle curve, convex anteriorly, should be formed by a line drawn along the tips of the spinous processes from C-2 to C-7 (dotted line 4).

Constructing these four lines on the lateral view of the cervical spine can be most helpful in assessing alignment of the vertebrae and in detecting any impingement upon the spinal canal. Which two of the four contour lines outline the anterior and posterior margins of the spinal canal? Of course, line 2 and line 3 do. If you scrutinize line 2, you will see that the anterior margin of the spinal canal is formed from the posterior margins of the cervical vertebral bodies and their intervening intervertebral discs. Line 3 outlines the posterior bony margin of the spinal canal, formed from the bases of the spinous processes. You must understand the bony boundaries of the spinal canal, as traumatic disruption of these boundaries or their ligamentous connections can result in serious damage to the spinal cord.

CHAPTER 3

NORMAL ANATOMY OF THE LATERAL MASSES, ARTICULAR PILLARS, LAMINAE, AND SPINOUS PROCESSES

Lateral Masses and Articular Pillars

The terms "lateral masses" and "articular pillars" are sometimes used synonymously. We will apply the term *lateral masses* to only the C-1 vertebra, or atlas. The term *articular pillars* will be applied to all the other cervical vertebrae.

Since the C-1 vertebra (the atlas) has no vertebral body, the main weight-bearing structures of C-1 are the lateral masses. These functionally replace the central vertebral body and, because of their location, are often referred to as the lateral masses of C-1. (These masses of bone make up the largest portion of the C-1 vertebra and appear as somewhat wedge-shaped structures on the anteroposterior projection of the C-1 vertebra; Fig. 4B.) On the lateral projection of the cervical spine, the lateral masses of C-1 are seen as osseous structures partially obscuring the odontoid process of C-2 (the axis). Superiorly, each lateral mass has an articular facet, or joint surface, through which it articulates with an occipital condyle. The lateral masses of C-1 (the atlas) are shown by the shaded areas in Figure 4.

The remainder of the cervical vertebrae have bodies and articulate above and below through articular pillars. These articular pillars appear as rhomboid-shaped structures, projecting downward and posteriorly from the vertebral bodies when viewed on the lateral radiograph of the cervical spine (Figs. 1, 2, and 5). Anteriorly, the articular pillars are joined to the vertebral bodies by the pedicles. Posteriorly, they serve as

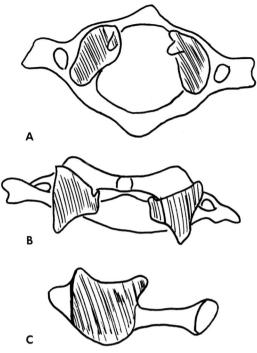

FIGURE 4

The C-1 vertebra, the atlas. *A*, As seen from above. *B*, As seen from the front (an anteroposterior projection). *C*, As seen from the side (a lateral projection). Shaded areas are the lateral masses.

the points of attachment for the laminae (Fig. 5). Together, the pedicles, articular pillars, and laminae make up the lateral and posterior bony margins of the spinal canal. The articular pillars are bounded above and below by the superior and inferior articular facets.

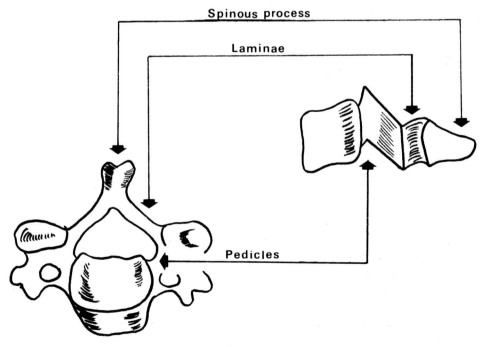

FIGURE 5

Laminae, pedicles, and spinous process of a cervical vertebra.

You will note that the inferior articular processes of one cervical vertebra lie behind the superior articular processes of the vertebra below it (Fig. 6). These articular processes have inclined surfaces which oppose each other, forming joint spaces. These joints are formed from bony processes and are often referred to as *apophyseal joints*. *Apophysis* is Greek for "an offshoot" and is used here to refer to the joints formed by the "offshoots" of the vertebrae that are the articular processes. For the purist, the term *zygapophyseal joints* may be used, as zygapophysis refers to the articular process of a vertebra. In any event, the inferior articular processes of C-4 articulate with the superior articular processes of C-5, forming the apophyseal joints. These joints are seen as radiolucent slits between the articular processes on the lateral cervical spine radiograph. Look at the lateral radiograph of the cervical spine and identify the apophyseal joint spaces (Fig. 1). The inclined surfaces of the articular processes help keep the vertebral bodies aligned and prevent them from sliding anteriorly over one another.

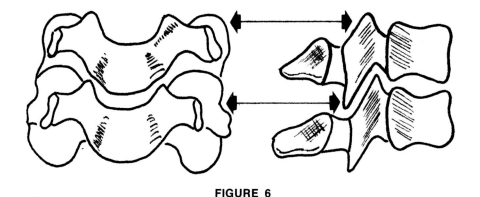

FIGURE 6

Apophyseal joints. In the frontal projection, these are not well seen. They can be readily identified on the lateral view.

In the anteroposterior projection of the cervical spine, the apophyseal joint spaces are not well seen. This should not surprise you when you recall the slope of the articular processes which form the margins of the apophyseal joints. Since the superior and inferior articular processes are inclined (Fig. 6), they are seen *en face* in the anteroposterior projection. In this view, therefore, when you look for the apophyseal joints, what you actually see are overlapping articular processes, and not the joint spaces.

You have now had an opportunity to view and review the anatomy of the articular pillars and to study their rhomboid configuration on the lateral radiograph of the cervical spine. What on earth are those double lines at the posterior margins of the rhomboids of C-4, C-5, and C-6 vertebrae in Figure 1? These parallel lines are often seen on lateral radiographs of the cervical spine and represent the posterior edges of the two articular processes, which are seldom perfectly superimposed. Figure 7A shows an imaginary radiographic beam traversing two perfectly superimposed articular processes of a vertebra. No double lines are seen at the posterior margin of the rhomboid formed by the articular processes. Figure 7B shows the path of radiographic beams traversing a vertebra in which the articular processes are not superimposed; in other words, a very slightly oblique projection. A double line is now apparent at the posterior margins of the rhomboids.

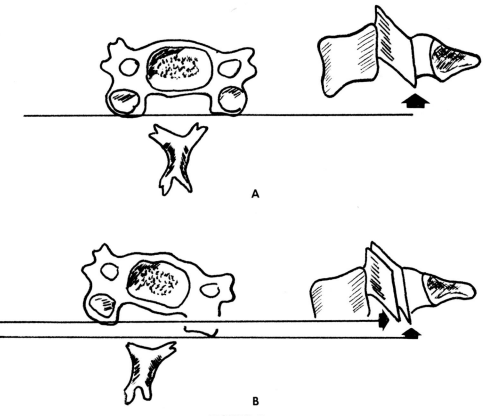

FIGURE 7
A, True lateral projection. B, Slightly oblique projection.

Laminae and Spinous Processes

The laminae project posteriorly to the articular pillars of the vertebrae and form a bony roof over the spinal canal. The laminae join in the midline, giving rise to the base of the spinous process (Fig. 8). On the lateral radiograph of the cervical spine, the bases of the spinous processes appear as white radiodense curved lines. Their convex surfaces face anteriorly and outline the posterior bony margin of the spinal canal. Find these radiodense curved lines on the lateral radiograph of the cervical spine (Fig. 1). Mentally join these lines together. They should form a smoothly contoured line, convex anteriorly, extending up and down the cervical spine. Any disruption in the smooth contour of this line, causing it to have a zigzag or "step-off" configuration, indicates a malalignment of the posterior bony margin of the spinal canal. The radiodense curved lines formed by the bases of the spinous processes not only mark the posterior bony boundary of the spinal canal, but also indicate the posterior margins of the laminae (Fig. 8). Since this radiodense curved line marks the bases of the spinous processes and posterior margins of the laminae, it is referred to as the *spinolaminal line* (Fig. 3, line 3).

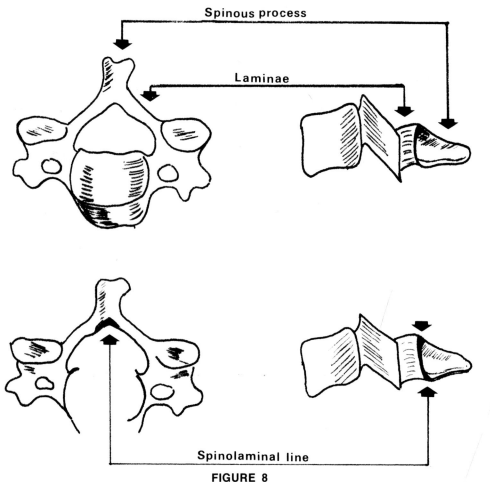

FIGURE 8
Spinous process, laminae, and the spinolaminal line.

CHAPTER 4

NORMAL ANATOMY OF THE OCCIPITO-ATLANTO-AXIAL JOINTS

Occipito-Atlanto-Axial Joints

Figure 9 shows diagrammatically the lateral (*A*) and anteroposterior (*B*) views of the occipito-atlanto-axial joints.

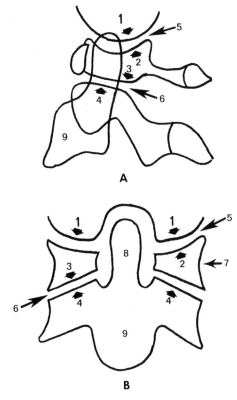

FIGURE 9
Occipito-atlanto-axial joints. *A*, Lateral view. *B*, Anteroposterior view.
1. Articular surface of occipital condyles
2. Superior articular facet of C-1
3. Inferior articular facet of C-1
4. Superior articular facet of C-2
5. Occipito-atlantal joint
6. Atlanto-axial joint
7. Lateral mass of C-1
8. Odontoid process
9. Body of C-2

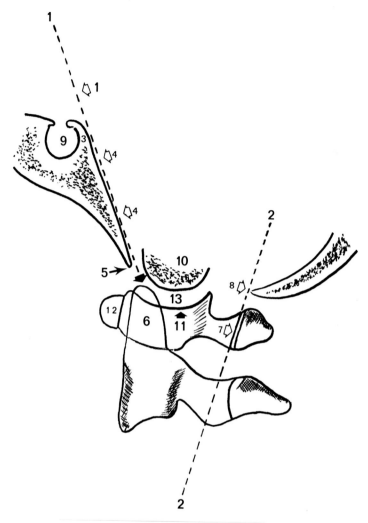

FIGURE 10

Lateral view of the occipito-atlanto-axial joints.
1. Line drawn from the dorsum sellae to anterior margin of the foramen magnum extends down the clivus and points to the odontoid process
2. Line drawn tangential to the spinolaminal surface of C-1 points to the posterior margin of the foramen magnum
3. Dorsum sellae
4. Clivus
5. Anterior margin of foramen magnum
6. Odontoid process
7. Spinolaminal surface of C-1
8. Posterior margin of foramen magnum
9. Sella turcica
10. Occipital condyle
11. Superior articular facet of C-1
12. Anterior arch of C-1
13. Occipito-atlantal joint

The occipito-atlantal joints are formed from the occipital condyles resting upon the superior articular facets of C-1. This can be seen on the lateral radiograph of the cervical spine. Often the tips of the mastoid processes of the temporal bone obscure the occipital condyles, making determination of alignment difficult. To avoid this problem, two other landmarks may be used to evaluate the alignment of the occipito-atlantal joints. These landmarks relate the anterior margin of the foramen magnum to the odontoid process and the posterior margin of the foramen magnum to the base of the spinous process of C-1 (lines 1 and 2, Fig. 10).

First, identify the anterior margin of the foramen magnum. This is done by projecting a line downward from the dorsum sellae, along the clivus (the bony plane formed from the fusion of the sphenoid bone with the occipital bone) to the anterior bony margin of the foramen magnum (line 1, Fig. 10). This line must point to or pass through the tip of the odontoid process. Normally, therefore, the tip of the odontoid points to the anterior edge of the foramen magnum. It is important to note that this line may be abnormal when there is a displaced fracture of the odontoid or an atlanto-axial subluxation.

A second line, drawn tangential to the spinolaminal surface of the posterior arch of C-1, should point to the posterior margin of the foramen magnum (Fig. 10). The posterior margin of the foramen magnum is identified as a beak-shaped or pointed edge where the inner table and outer table of the occipital bone merge. When these two lines are correctly oriented, the occipito-atlantal joints can be said to be in normal alignment on the lateral radiograph of the cervical spine.

The two occipito-atlantal joints just described allow the head to flex on the atlas. This movement allows you to express a "yes" or to check if your fly is open. Flexion and extension of the head on the remainder of the cervical spine occur at the occipito-atlantal joints. Rotation of the head on the remainder of the cervical spine occurs at the atlanto-axial joints.

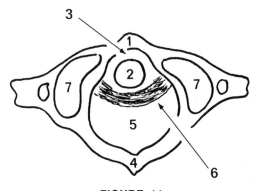

FIGURE 11
Bird's eye view of the atlanto-axial joint.
1. Anterior arch of atlas
2. Odontoid process
3. Space between the anterior arch of atlas and the odontoid process
4. Posterior arch of the atlas
5. Spinal canal
6. Transverse ligament
7. Superior articular facets of atlas

The anterior arch of C-1 is fixed in relation to the odontoid process of C-2 by the transverse ligament (Fig. 11). This ligament is attached to the lateral masses of C-1. Two joints are thus formed. One joint is formed between the posterior surface of the anterior arch of C-1 and the anterior surface of the odontoid process. A second joint occurs between the posterior surface of the odontoid and the anterior surface of the transverse ligament of C-1 (Fig. 11). These two joints, together with the joints formed between the inferior articular facets of C-1 and the superior articular facets of C-2, compose the four atlanto-axial joints (Fig. 9).

The names of the vertebrae forming the atlanto-axial joints can be hard to remember. Think of the head as the world being supported by the C-1 vertebra, which is named after the Greek god Atlas.

The C-2 vertebra is more complex because of the bony process which projects upward from the anterior surface of its vertebral body. This bony process is commonly called the odontoid process, but it may also be referred to as the dens. Interestingly enough, both names refer to teeth. Odontoid comes from the Greek word *odous*, meaning "tooth," while dens comes from the Latin word *dens*, also meaning "tooth." Axis, the name for the C-2 vertebra, is easy to remember. Think of it as the axis about which the atlas turns.

In evaluating the atlanto-axial joint, the distance separating the anterior arch of the atlas (C-1) from the odontoid process should be examined carefully (Fig. 12). This distance in the adult should not exceed 2.5 mm. even when the head is flexed on the cervical spine, as the transverse ligament of the atlas keeps the anterior arch of the atlas firmly fixed against the odontoid process. Any increase in this space indicates forward displacement of the atlas on the axis and is abnormal. In children, with flexion of the head, the atlas normally moves forward on the axis, and the space between the anterior arch of the atlas and odontoid process may normally increase to 5 mm. A space wider than 5 mm. is abnormal.

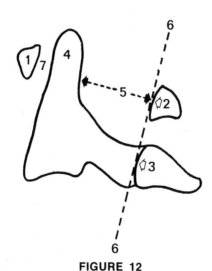

FIGURE 12

Lateral view of the atlanto-axial joint.
1. Anterior arch of atlas
2. Base of spinous process of C-1
3. Base of spinous process of C-2
4. Odontoid process
5. Dotted line showing the sagittal diameter of the spinal canal at the level of the atlanto-axial joint
6. Dotted line showing the normal contour of the bases of the spinous processes of C-1 and C-2
7. Space between the anterior arch of the atlas and the odontoid process

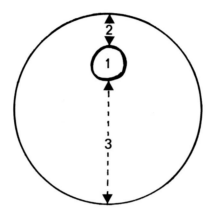

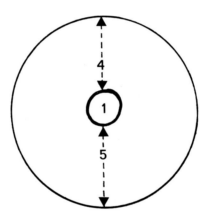

FIGURE 13
Ring diagram of the atlanto-axial joint as seen from above.
1. Odontoid process
2. Normal narrow distance between the anterior ring and odontoid process
3. Normal wide distance between posterior ring and odontoid process
4. Abnormally wide distance between anterior ring and odontoid process
5. Abnormally narrow distance between posterior ring and odontoid process, compromising spinal canal

Special attention should be paid to the sagittal diameter of the spinal canal at the level of the atlanto-axial joint (Fig. 13). When the space between the anterior arch of the atlas and the odontoid process widens, the space between the posterior arch of the atlas and the odontoid process must decrease. This is only natural, since the atlas is simply a ring.

When the space between the posterior arch of the atlas and the odontoid process narrows, the sagittal diameter of the spinal canal is compromised at that level. The sagittal diameter of the spinal canal is the shortest distance between the posterior border of a vertebral body and the base of a spinous process (Fig. 12). When one examines the spinal cord at the autopsy table and sees that its anteroposterior diameter is approximately 1 cm., it is not hard to understand why a sagittal diameter of less than 12 mm. will compress the cord at any level. To appreciate narrowing of the sagittal diameter of the spinal canal, measurements can be made directly from lateral radiographs of the cervical spine if these radiographs do not show significant magnification. Narrowing of the space between the posterior arch of the atlas and the odontoid process can also be detected by observing a "step-off" or zigzag configuration in a line drawn parallel to the spinolaminal surfaces of the atlas and the axis. The dotted line in Figure 12 shows the normal contour of the bases of the spinous processes of the atlas and axis.

CHAPTER 5
NORMAL ANATOMY OF THE CERVICAL LIGAMENTS AND SOFT TISSUES

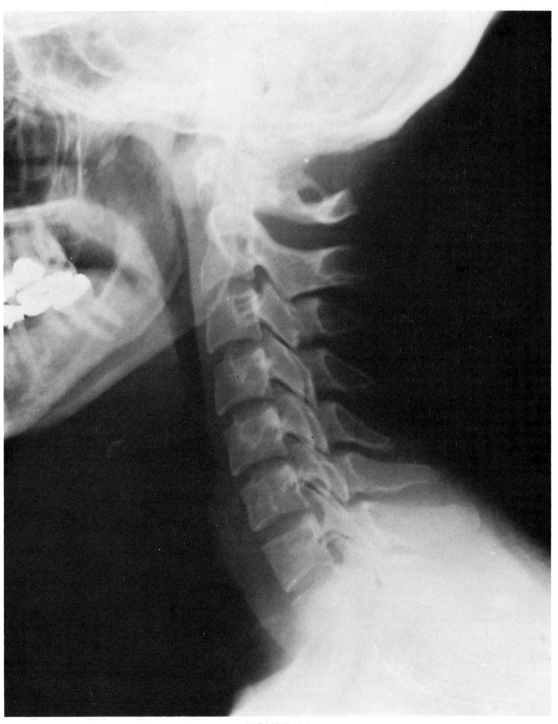

FIGURE 14

Can you identify the location of each of the ligamentous structures listed below and relate them to the osseous structures seen on the lateral radiograph of the cervical spine (Fig. 14) on the opposite page?

1. Anterior longitudinal ligament

2. Posterior longitudinal ligament

3. Capsular ligaments

4. Ligamenta flava

5. Interspinous ligaments

6. Ligamentum nuchae*

7. Supraspinous ligament

*The ligamentum nuchae includes the supraspinous ligament and the fibers that form the interspinous ligaments.

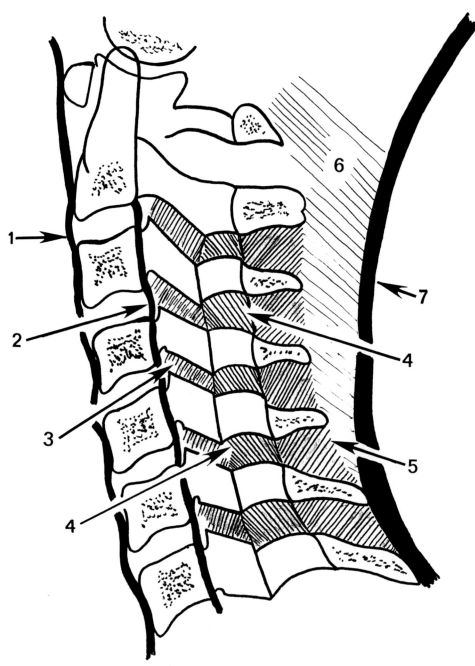

FIGURE 15

Name the anatomic structures numbered on the diagram (Fig. 15) of the lateral radiograph of the cervical spine on the opposite page.

1. _____

   _____

2. _____

   _____

3. _____

   _____

4. _____

   _____

5. _____

   _____

6. _____

   _____

7. _____

   _____

We hope you've caught on by now that the correct answers are listed on the previous page. We're sure you got them all right.

Ligamentous Anatomy

The major ligaments of the cervical spine are the anterior longitudinal ligament, the posterior longitudinal ligament, the capsular ligaments, the ligamenta flava, and the ligamentum nuchae (the interspinous and supraspinous ligaments).

The anterior longitudinal ligament is a strong narrow band of dense fibrous connective tissue which extends from the clivus to the sacrum. It is attached to the anterior margins of the vertebral bodies and the intervertebral discs (Fig. 16).

The posterior longitudinal ligament is located within the bony spinal canal. It begins at the posterior surface of C-2 and continues down to the sacrum. It hugs the posterior aspects of the vertebral bodies and fans out slightly over the intervertebral discs (Fig. 16).

The capsular ligaments surround the zygapophyseal joints of the cervical spine, between the superior and inferior articular processes (Fig. 17A). The capsular ligaments have some laxity.

The ligamenta flava are composed of elastic tissue and connect the laminae of adjacent vertebrae (Figs. 17B and 18). Elastic in nature, they permit separation of the laminae during flexion.

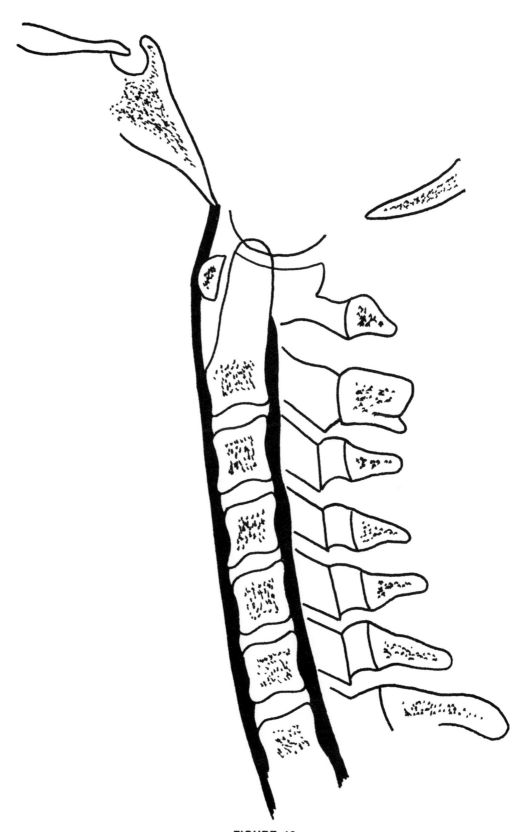

FIGURE 16
The anterior and posterior longitudinal ligaments

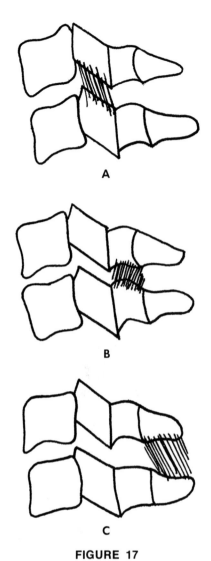

FIGURE 17

A, The capsular ligaments; *B*, the ligamenta flava; and *C*, the interspinous ligaments.

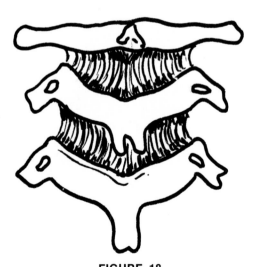

FIGURE 18

The ligamenta flava as seen from behind

The ligamentum nuchae is a complex structure (Fig. 19). It is fan-shaped and extends superiorly from the region of the external occipital protuberance to the region of the foramen magnum. It then continues inferiorly. In its course, this ligament gives off fibers which pass between the spinous processes to form the interspinous ligaments (Figs. 17C and 19).

The posterior margin of the ligamentum nuchae forms the supra-spinous ligament (Fig. 19). The tips of the spinous processes of the C-6 and C-7 vertebrae are directly attached to the supraspinous ligament. The tips of the other cervical spinous processes are not directly attached to the supraspinous ligament.

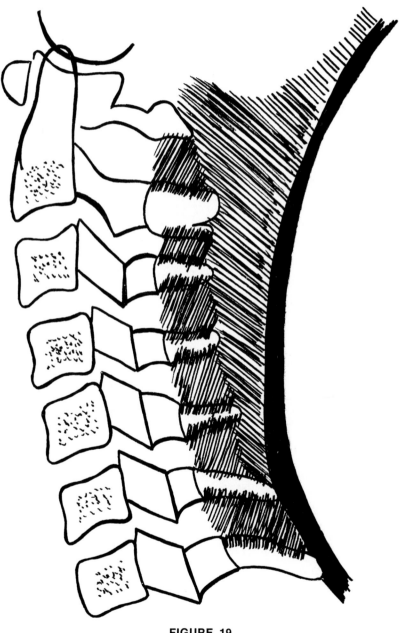

FIGURE 19
The ligamentum nuchae

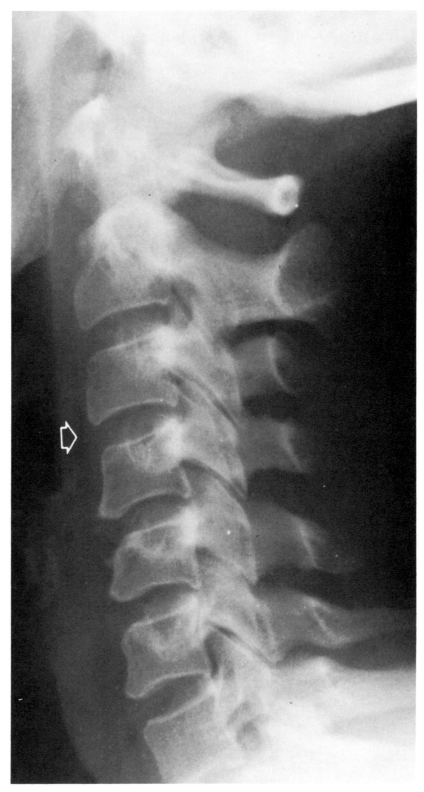

FIGURE 20
The prevertebral fat stripe

In the prevertebral soft tissues in the upper and mid-cervical regions, a radiolucent fat stripe may be identified. This fat stripe parallels the anterior margins of the vertebral bodies (Fig. 20). The location of this structure should be checked carefully in all cases of suspected trauma, and localized displacements should be noted.

Many of the lateral radiographs of patients with neck trauma are made with some magnification, due to the cross-table technique. Thus, only relative measurements of the prevertebral soft tissues can be made. As a general rule, in adults the prevertebral tissues should not exceed four-tenths of the anteroposterior diameter of the vertebral body of C-4. This measurement is made between the air column and the anterior bony margin of the vertebra.

CHAPTER 6

TEST CASES 1 AND 2

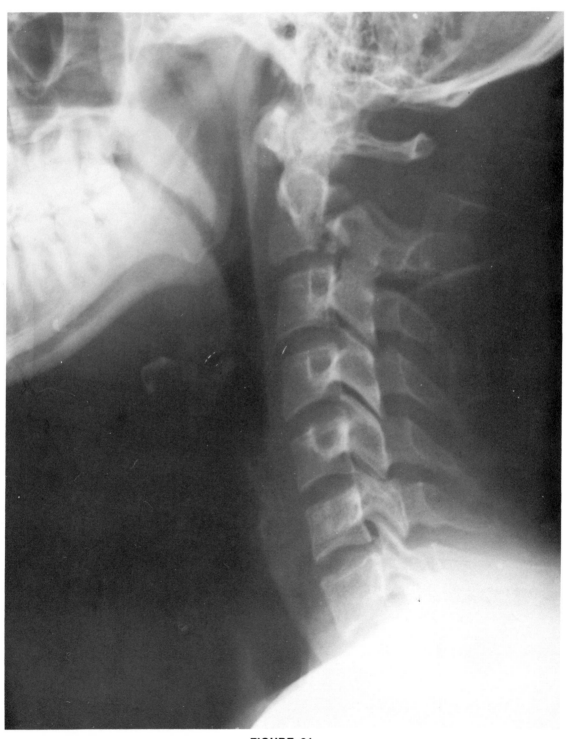

FIGURE 21
Test Case 1

TEST CASE 1

WHAT IS YOUR DIAGNOSIS?

1. Which anatomic structure or structures are involved? _____

   _____

   _____

2. Are the involved structures displaced or nondisplaced? _____

   _____

   _____

3. Is this a stable or an unstable injury? _____

   _____

   _____

4. What is the common eponym or diagnostic term for the type of injury
   seen on the radiograph? _____

   _____

   _____

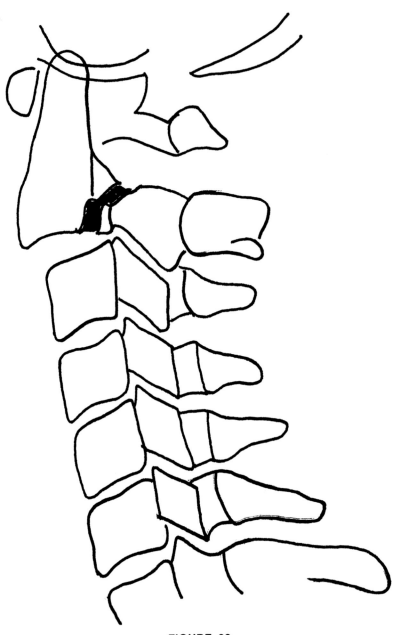

FIGURE 22
Test Case 1

TEST CASE 1

ANSWERS:

1. Which anatomic structure or structures are involved? *Fractures of both pedicles of C-2; fracture of the posterior inferior margin of the C-2 vertebral body*

2. Are the involved structures displaced or nondisplaced? *The C-2 vertebral body is displaced slightly anteriorly on the C-3 vertebral body.*

3. Is this a stable or an unstable injury? *Unstable*

4. What is the common eponym or diagnostic term for the type of injury seen on the radiograph? *Hangman's fracture*

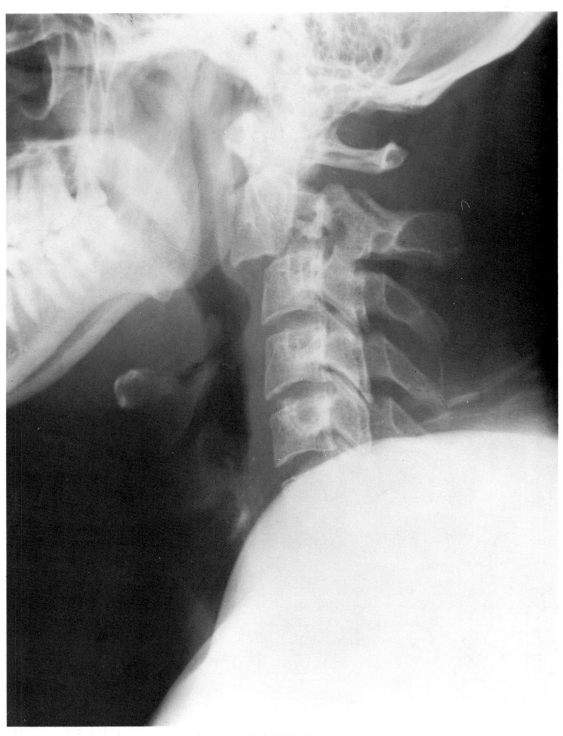

FIGURE 23
Test Case 2

TEST CASE 2

WHAT IS YOUR DIAGNOSIS?

1. Which anatomic structure or structures are involved? _____

_____

_____

2. Are the involved structures displaced or nondisplaced? _____

_____

_____

3. Is this a stable or an unstable injury? _____

_____

_____

4. What is the common eponym or diagnostic term for the type of injury seen on the radiograph? _____

_____

_____

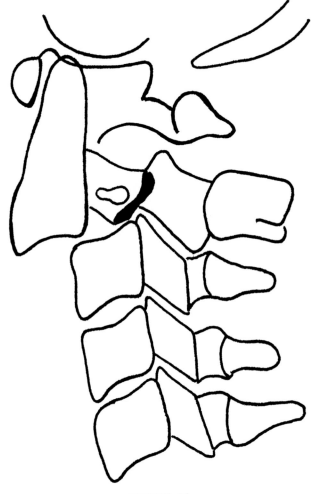

FIGURE 24
Test Case 2

TEST CASE 2

ANSWERS:

1. Which anatomic structure or structures are involved? *Bilateral pedicle fractures of C-2; torn anterior and posterior longitudinal ligaments*

2. Are the involved structures displaced or nondisplaced? *Forward displacement of the vertebral body of the axis (C-2) on the vertebral body of C-3*

3. Is this a stable or an unstable injury? *Unstable*

4. What is the common eponym or diagnostic term for the type of injury seen on the radiograph? *Hangman's fracture*

The Hangman's Fracture

Since this fracture is identical to those created by judicial hangings, it has been called the "hangman's fracture." Actually, when you think about it, it is not the "hangman" who is fractured, but rather the "hang-ee." So, why not call this fracture the "hangee fracture"? In any event, the mechanism of injury is hyperextension of the head on the neck. This injury, nowadays, occurs in an auto accident when the chin or forehead hits the steering wheel or dashboard, forcing the head into hyperextension. Think of this fracture as resulting from displacement of the C-2 vertebral body upward and the inferior articular facets of C-2 downward. The result is a fracture through the pedicles of C-2. The fracture lines lie anterior to the inferior articular facets of C-2 and posterior to the superior articular facets of C-2 (Fig. 25). Since both pedicles are fractured, there is no bony support to keep the C-2 vertebral body from slipping forward on the C-3 vertebral body, and it usually does (Figs. 21 and 23). The inferior articular facets of C-2 remain in their normal location, and the apophyseal joints between the inferior articular facets of C-2 and the superior articular facets of C-3 remain relatively intact. Note that in both Figure 21 and Figure 23, the spinolaminal surface or base of the spinous process of C-2 has not moved forward and the spinolaminal line remains intact from the C-2 level downward. In other words, no "step-off" is pres-

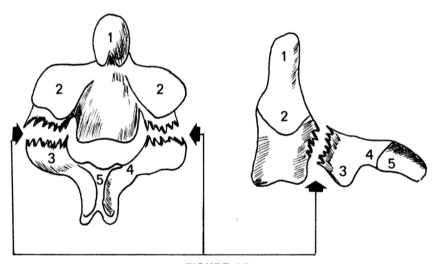

FIGURE 25

Hangman's fracture. The arrows point to the fractures through the pedicles anterior to the inferior articular facets and posterior to the superior articular facets.
1. Odontoid process
2. Superior articular facets
3. Inferior articular facets
4. Laminae
5. Spinous process

ent between the base of the spinous process of C-2 and the base of the spinous process of C-3. The spinolaminal line is disrupted between the base of the spinous process of C-2 and the posterior arch of C-1. This disruption is seen especially well in Figure 23 and is the result of the posterior arch of C-1 slipping anterior to the base of the spinous process of C-2. This occurs because as the body of C-2 slips forward on the body of C-3, it carries with it the odontoid process. The odontoid process pulls the anterior arch of C-1 forward as well as its posterior arch. What else is displaced anteriorly? The answer is the skull, of course! Since the occipito-atlanto-axial joints are preserved in this injury, the skull, the entire C-1 vertebra, the odontoid process, and the body of C-2 can be considered to be displaced forward on the remainder of the cervical spine.

Summary of the Radiographic Findings of Hangman's Fracture

1. Hangman's fractures are best seen on lateral radiographs of the cervical spine.
2. The occipito-atlanto-axial joints and odontoid process are intact.
3. The bilateral pedicle fractures of C-2 are anterior to the inferior articular facets.
4. The C-2 vertebral body is often displaced anterior to the vertebral body of C-3.

CHAPTER 7
TEST CASES 3, 4, AND 5

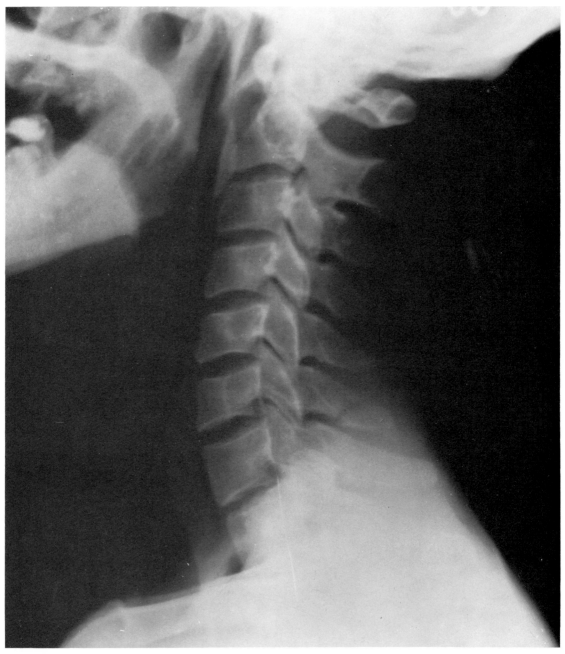

FIGURE 26
Test Case 3

TEST CASE 3

WHAT IS YOUR DIAGNOSIS?

1. Which anatomic structure or structures are involved? _____

_____

_____

2. Are the involved structures displaced or nondisplaced? _____

_____

_____

3. Is this a stable or an unstable injury? _____

_____

_____

4. What is the common eponym or diagnostic term for the type of injury seen on the radiograph? _____

_____

_____

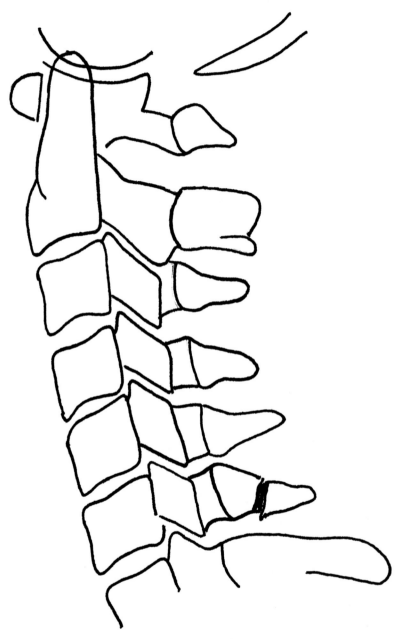

FIGURE 27
Test Case 3

ANSWERS:

1. Which anatomic structure or structures are involved? *Spinous process of the C-6 vertebra*

2. Are the involved structures displaced or nondisplaced? *Inferior displacement of the tip of the spinous process*

3. Is this a stable or an unstable injury? *Stable*

4. What is the common eponym or diagnostic term for the type of injury seen on the radiograph? *Clay shoveler's fracture*

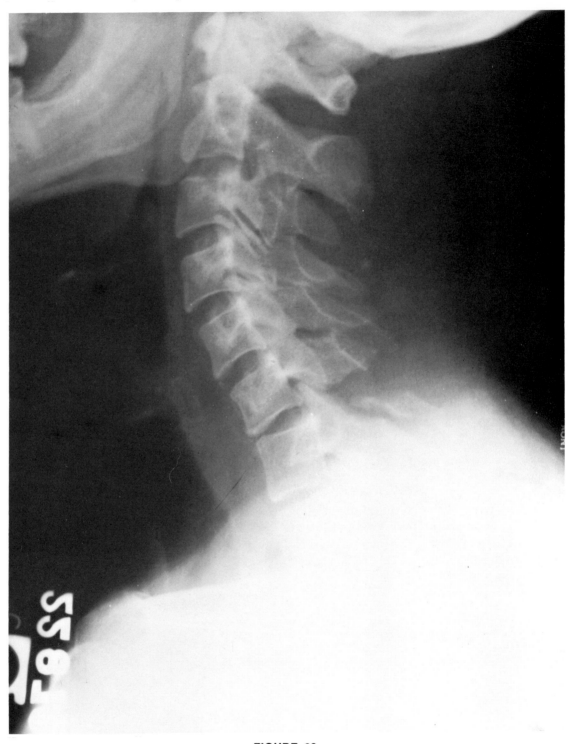

FIGURE 28
Test Case 4

TEST CASE 4

WHAT IS YOUR DIAGNOSIS?

1. Which anatomic structure or structures are involved? _____

_____

_____

2. Are the involved structures displaced or nondisplaced? _____

_____

_____

3. Is this a stable or an unstable injury? _____

_____

_____

4. What is the common eponym or diagnostic term for the type of injury seen on the radiograph? _____

_____

_____

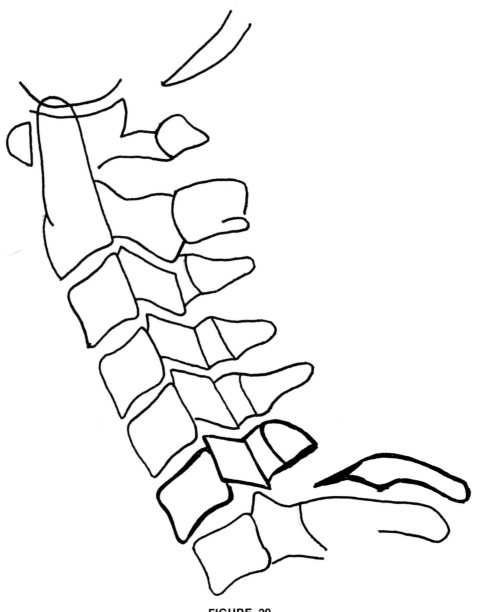

FIGURE 29
Test Case 4

TEST CASE 4

ANSWERS:

1. Which anatomic structure or structures are involved? *Spinous process and inferior aspect of the lamina of the C-6 vertebra. Also, the interspinous and supraspinous ligaments are torn.*

2. Are the involved structures displaced or nondisplaced? *Spinous process and inferior aspect of the lamina of the C-6 vertebra are displaced downward. There is superior displacement of the inferior articular facet of C-6 on the superior articular facet of C-7. This has caused the vertebral body of C-6 to be tilted forward.*

3. Is this a stable or an unstable injury? *Unstable (Patient may be transported in extension with care.)*

4. What is the common eponym or diagnostic term for the type of injury seen on the radiograph? *Clay shoveler's fracture*

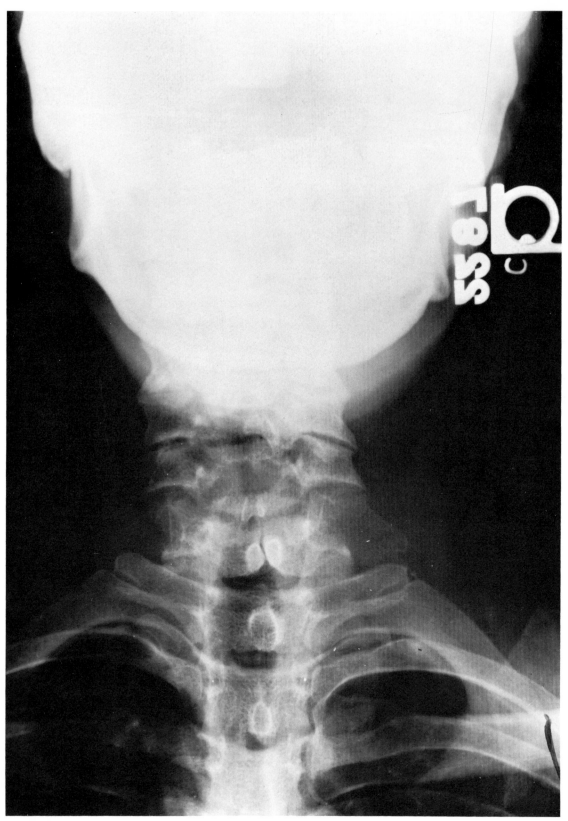

FIGURE 30
Test Case 5

TEST CASE 5

WHAT IS YOUR DIAGNOSIS?

1. Which anatomic structure or structures are involved? _____

_____

_____

2. Are the involved structures displaced or nondisplaced? _____

_____

_____

3. Is this a stable or an unstable injury? _____

_____

_____

4. What is the common eponym or diagnostic term for the type of injury seen on the radiograph? _____

_____

_____

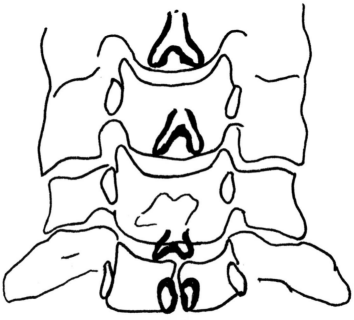

FIGURE 31
Test Case 5

TEST CASE 5

ANSWERS:

1. Which anatomic structure or structures are involved? *Spinous process and inferior aspect of the lamina of the C-6 vertebra. (This is the anteroposterior view of the cervical spine seen in Test Case 4.)*

2. Are the involved structures displaced or nondisplaced? *Inferior displacement of the spinous process and inferior aspect of the lamina of the C-6 vertebra.*

3. Is this a stable or an unstable injury? *Unstable (See Test Case 4.)*

4. What is the common eponym or diagnostic term for the type of injury seen on the radiograph? *Clay shoveler's fracture*

(Were you troubled by the appearance of the C-7 laminae and spinous process? This patient has incomplete bony fusion of the posterior neural arch, a normal anatomic variant.)

The Clay Shoveler's Fracture

The term "clay shoveler's fracture" was coined in Germany, where the injury was seen among workers employed in building the Autobahn. Everything was fine as long as it didn't rain and the beer flowed freely. However, when it rained these poor fellows were driven out to work in the wet. Their spirits were dampened, as was the soil, which became mighty heavy. A fantastic force was transmitted to the spinous processes of the lower neck by the thoracoscapular muscles as the men heaved clay into trucks. As these workers lifted shovels full of wet and heavy clay, they sustained avulsion fractures of the spinous processes of the lower cervical and upper thoracic spine. The fractures usually occurred at C-6, C-7, or T-1 and occasionally at T-2.

So you say you don't shovel clay. You can still get this fracture! A modern-day counterpart to this injury is seen after many a poolroom brawl. Direct trauma to spinous processes, such as a blow on the back of the neck by a pool cue, can also cause this injury.

Indirect trauma to the neck in car accidents can also result in fractures of the spinous processes. The mechanism of injury in this case is a sudden hyperflexion of the head on the neck. This causes a sudden pull on the ligamentum nuchae, the interspinous and supraspinous ligaments. Since the supraspinous ligament is directly attached to the tips of the spinous processes of C-6 and C-7, avulsion fractures of these spinous processes occur with tearing of the supraspinous ligament.

Tears of the major cervical ligaments can allow the spinous processes to separate, resulting in vertebral body displacement and malalignment of the apophyseal joints (Fig. 28).

Fractures of the spinous processes of C-6 and C-7 vertebrae may not be seen on underexposed lateral roentgenograms. This is particularly true in patients with short, thick necks or wide shoulders. When such a fracture is present, the anteroposterior view will show inferior displacement of the tip of the spinous process and will show an abnormally wide space between the visualized spinous processes.

Summary of the Radiographic Findings in Clay Shoveler's Fracture

1. Clay shoveler's fractures are best seen on the lateral radiograph of the cervical spine and most commonly involve the spinous processes of C-6 and C-7.
2. The tip of the fractured spinous process is frequently displaced inferiorly.
3. An abnormal contour and position of the spinous process may be noted on the anteroposterior radiograph.
4. Associated ligamentous tears may accompany this fracture and may permit malalignment of the apophyseal joints.

CHAPTER 8

TEST CASES 6 AND 7

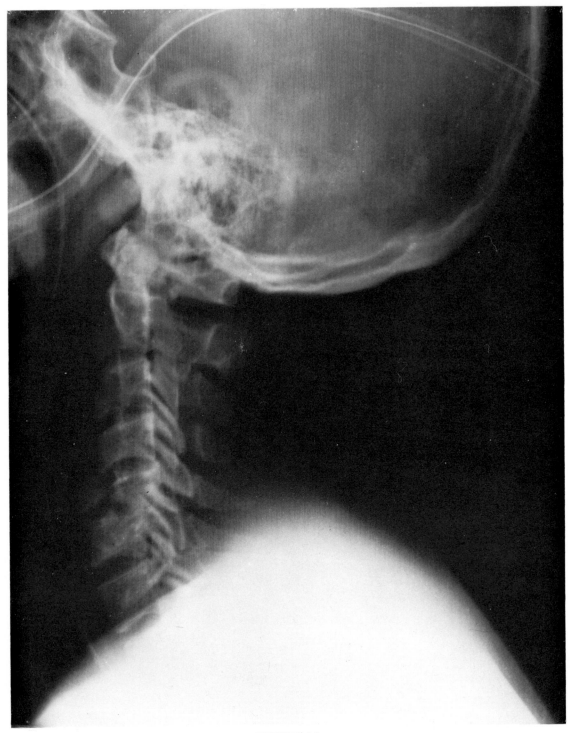

FIGURE 32
Test Case 6

TEST CASE 6

WHAT IS YOUR DIAGNOSIS?

1. Which anatomic structure or structures are involved? _____

   _____

   _____

2. Are the involved structures displaced or nondisplaced? _____

   _____

   _____

3. Is this a stable or an unstable injury? _____

   _____

   _____

4. What is the common eponym or diagnostic term for the type of injury
   seen on the radiograph? _____

   _____

   _____

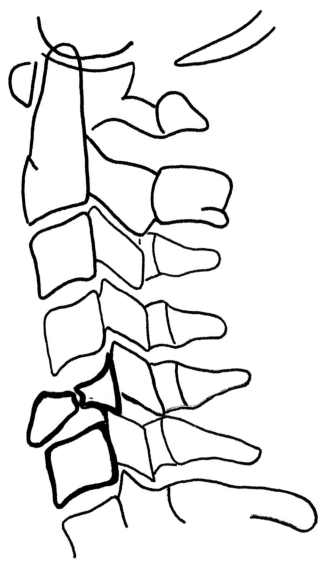

FIGURE 33
Test Case 6

TEST CASE 6

ANSWERS:

1. Which anatomic structure or structures are involved? *Fragmented compression fracture of the C-5 vertebral body*

2. Are the involved structures displaced or nondisplaced? *Posterior displacement of the fractured C-5 vertebral body with narrowing of the spinal canal. There is disruption of the spinolaminal line at C-5 and C-6.*

3. Is this a stable or an unstable injury? *Stable (There is a high probability of spinal cord damage due to posterior displacement of fracture fragments and disc material.)*

4. What is the common eponym or diagnostic term for the type of injury seen on the radiograph? *Bursting or compression fracture*

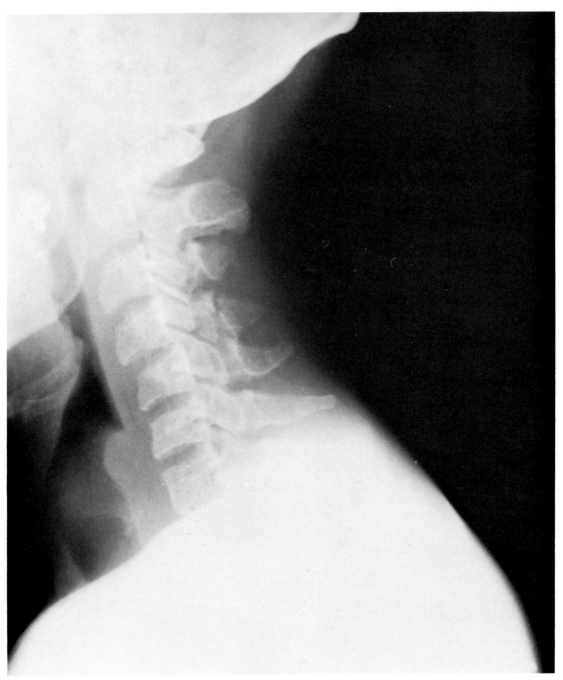

FIGURE 34
Test Case 7

TEST CASE 7

WHAT IS YOUR DIAGNOSIS?

1. Which anatomic structure or structures are involved? _____

_____

_____

2. Are the involved structures displaced or nondisplaced? _____

_____

_____

3. Is this a stable or an unstable injury? _____

_____

_____

4. What is the common eponym or diagnostic term for the type of injury seen on the radiograph? _____

_____

_____

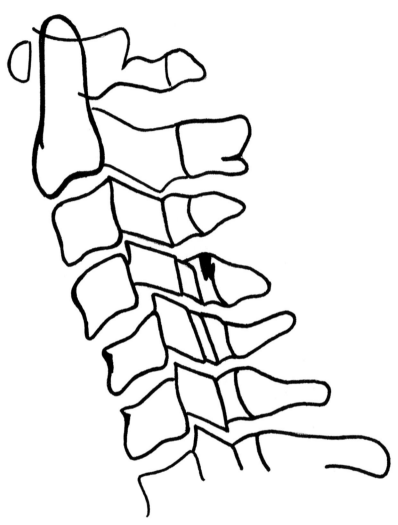

FIGURE 35
Test Case 7

TEST CASE 7

ANSWERS:

1. Which anatomic structure or structures are involved? *Laminae and base of the spinous process of C-4. Anterior wedging compression fractures of the C-5 and C-6 vertebral bodies are also present.*

2. Are the involved structures displaced or nondisplaced? *C-4 vertebral body is anteriorly displaced on the C-5 vertebral body.*

3. Is this a stable or an unstable injury? *Unstable, because of the fractures through the posterior neural arch*

4. What is the common eponym or diagnostic term for the type of injury seen on the radiograph? *Compression fractures with posterior element fractures*

Vertebral Body Compression Fracture

Vertebral body compression fractures occur through two different mechanisms. Test Case 6 illustrates the first of these mechanisms. When severe opposing forces are applied to the long axis of the cervical spine, a "bursting" compression fracture results. Figure 36 shows the opposing lines of force causing the C-4 and C-6 vertebral bodies to come together, sandwiching C-5 in the middle. The result is self-evident—fragmentation of the body of C-5.

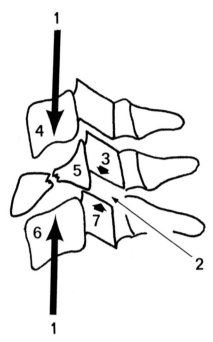

FIGURE 36
The mechanism of injury in a bursting compression fracture.
1. Lines of forces along the axis of the cervical spine compressing the C-5 vertebral body between C-4 and C-6
2. Widened apophyseal joint space between C-5 and C-6
3. Inferior articular facets of C-5
4. C-4 vertebral body
5. Posteriorly displaced fracture fragment of the C-5 vertebral body
6. C-6 vertebral body
7. Superior articular facet of C-6

Note that in Test Case 6 the anterior part of the C-5 vertebral body has been driven forward, causing a zigzag configuration of the anterior contour line of the cervical spine (Fig. 32). Also, a portion of the vertebral body is displaced posteriorly. This can be seen on the lateral radiograph of the cervical spine as a "step-off" in the contour line drawn down the posterior margins of the vertebral bodies (Fig. 32). There is a significant decrease in the anteroposterior diameter of the spinal canal between the posterior fragment of C-5 and the base of the spinous process of C-6. It is this encroachment on the spinal canal that makes this fracture so dangerous. Careful analysis of the contour lines makes it easy to appreciate this encroachment.

The posterior displacement of the posterior fragment of the C-5 vertebral body in Test Case 6 has also caused the apophyseal joint space between the inferior articular facets of C-5 and the superior articular facets of C-6 to become wider. This has happened because the bony fragment carried with it its attached articular facets. Notice that all the vertebral bodies above the level of the fracture site are in alignment. Alignment is maintained because the displaced superior articular facets of the fractured C-5 vertebral body carried with them all the articular facets above this level. The result is that the entire cervical spine above the level of the fracture site at C-5 is posteriorly displaced with respect to the cervical spine below the level of the fracture. This displacement has also caused the base of the spinous process of C-5 to be positioned slightly behind the base of the spinous process of C-6. A "step-off" in the contour line drawn adjacent to these spinolaminal surfaces results (Figs. 32 and 37).

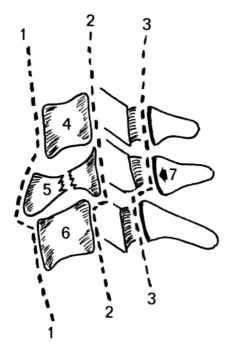

FIGURE 37

Malalignment produced by a bursting compression fracture of C-5.
1. Line 1 shows a zigzag configuration at the anterior surfaces of the C-4, C-5, and C-6 vertebral bodies.
2. Line 2 demonstrates a "step-off" configuration at the posterior surfaces of the C-5 and C-6 vertebral bodies.
3. Line 3 demonstrates a "step-off" configuration between the base of the spinous processes of C-5 and C-6.
4. C-4 vertebral body
5. Fractured C-5 vertebral body
6. C-6 vertebral body
7. Base of the spinous process of C-5

The second type of compression fracture of the cervical spine occurs as a result of a flexion injury. This type of injury is illustrated in Test Case 7. The lateral radiograph of the cervical spine in Figure 34 shows compression fractures of the anterior margins of the C-5 and C-6 vertebral bodies. Note that C-4 is displaced forward on C-5.

Now let's turn our attention to the fractures of the laminae and the base of the spinous process of the C-4 vertebra in Test Case 7 (Figs. 34 and 35). Forward flexion of the cervical spine separates the laminae and spinous processes of adjacent vertebral bodies. As the posterior arch is spread apart, the pulling forces of the interconnecting ligamenta flava and interspinous ligaments serve to keep the laminae and spinous processes in alignment. If these ligamentous structures are stressed, as occurs with forced flexion of the neck, the ligaments can tear and the bony structures to which they are attached may fracture, as in this test case (Figs. 34 and 38).

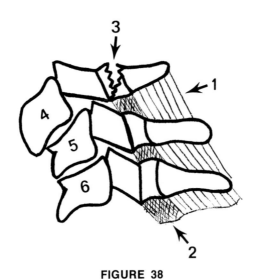

FIGURE 38

Mechanism of the laminae and spinous process fractures associated with vertebral body compression.

1. Interspinous ligament
2. Ligamenta flava
3. Fracture through the laminae and base of the spinous process of the C-4 vertebra
4. Vertebral body of C-4
5. Compressed vertebral body of C-5
6. Compressed vertebral body of C-6

You must remember that vertebral compression fractures vary widely in severity from minimal anterior wedging to complete disruption of the involved vertebral body. Once you have identified a compression fracture, you must also remember to look carefully for associated injuries, such as fractures of the pedicles, articular facets, laminae, and spinous processes.

Summary of the Radiographic Findings in Vertebral Compression Fractures

1. Vertebral compression fractures are best seen on the lateral radiograph of the cervical spine and are recognized by the loss of vertical height of the vertebral body.
2. Vertebral compression fractures may result either from flexion of the cervical spine or from compression forces applied to the long axis of the cervical spine.
3. Serious injury to the spinal cord may occur in association with compression fractures if there is encroachment on the spinal canal by displaced vertebral body or disc fragments or by associated hemorrhage.
4. Compression fractures of the cervical vertebrae may be associated with widening of the apophyseal joints and with fractures of the posterior vertebral arches.

CHAPTER 9
TEST CASE 8

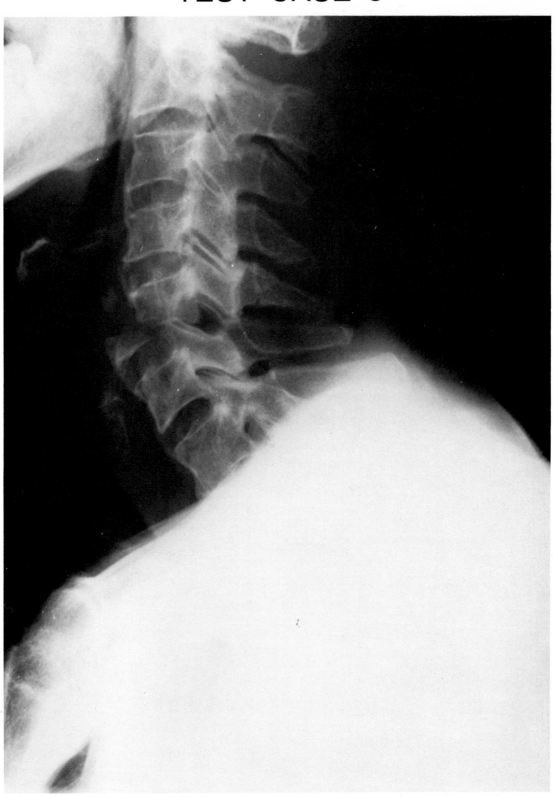

FIGURE 39
Test Case 8

TEST CASE 8

WHAT IS YOUR DIAGNOSIS?

1. Which anatomic structure or structures are involved? _____

   _____

   _____

2. Are the involved structures displaced or nondisplaced? _____

   _____

   _____

3. Is this a stable or an unstable injury? _____

   _____

   _____

4. What is the common eponym or diagnostic term for the type of injury
   seen on the radiograph? _____

   _____

   _____

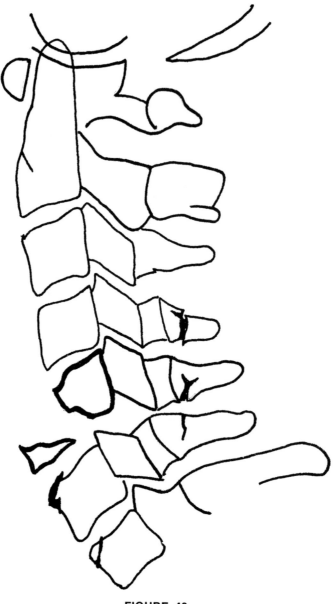

FIGURE 40
Test Case 8

TEST CASE 8

ANSWERS:

1. Which anatomic structure or structures are involved? *Large chip ("teardrop") avulsion fracture of the C-5 vertebral body and small nondisplaced avulsion fractures of the C-6 and C-7 vertebral bodies. The spinous processes of C-4, C-5, and C-6 are also fractured.*

2. Are the involved structures displaced or nondisplaced? *Posterior displacement of C-5 with respect to C-6. The spinal canal is narrowed.*

3. Is this a stable or an unstable injury? *Unstable*

4. What is the common eponym or diagnostic term for the type of injury seen on the radiograph? *Teardrop fracture*

Teardrop Fracture

Hyperextension injuries of the neck can cause chip fractures at the anterior margins of the vertebral bodies. With forceful hyperextension of the cervical spine, stress is applied to the anterior longitudinal ligament, which either ruptures or is avulsed from the vertebral bodies (Figs. 39 and 41). As this ligament is ruptured or pulled away from the surface of a vertebral body, it can take with it a piece of the anterior surface of that body. This small avulsed triangular piece of bone is shaped like a teardrop—in the minds of the imaginative—explaining why this is called a "teardrop fracture." These small teardrop fractures are an indication of the more serious soft tissue injuries due to hyperextension. Unfortunately, these serious injuries involving soft tissue structures are not seen on the radiograph. The traumatized soft tissues include the ligamenta flava, spinal cord, and anterior longitudinal ligament. Since we have already talked about the damage to the anterior longitudinal ligament, we will now turn our attention to injury of the ligamenta flava and spinal cord.

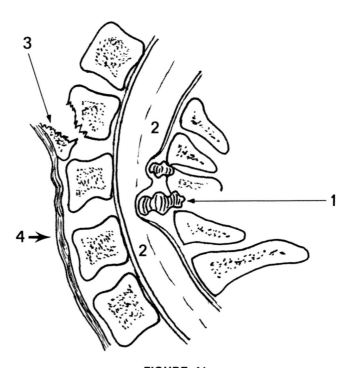

FIGURE 41
Contusion of the spinal cord by the ligamenta flava with a teardrop fracture.
1. Buckled ligamenta flava compressing the spinal cord
2. Spinal cord
3. The teardrop—an avulsed fracture fragment from the anterior margin of a vertebral body
4. Anterior longitudinal ligament

Figure 42 shows the ligamenta flava attached to the inner superior and inferior margins of the laminae. The laminae join in the midline at the spinous processes to form a roof over the spinal cord. With forceful hyperextension of the neck, the laminae are jammed together, causing the ligamenta flava to buckle inward into the spinal canal (Figure 41). This inward buckling of the compressed ligamenta flava compresses and contuses the spinal cord. You're in double jeopardy if the anteroposterior diameter of your spinal canal is congenitally small, or if old age has crept up on you and degenerative changes have narrowed your bony canal.

Teardrop fractures are unstable injuries. If the spinal cord is contused by buckling of the ligamenta flava at the time of impact, the neurologic manifestation is the so-called central spinal cord syndrome.

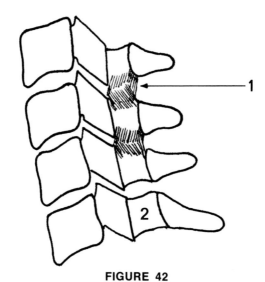

FIGURE 42
The attachment of the ligamenta flava to the inner margins of the laminae.
1. Ligamenta flava
2. Lamina of a cervical vertebra

Summary of Radiographic Findings in Teardrop Fractures

1. In the teardrop fracture, a triangular piece of vertebral body is seen in the soft tissues anterior to the vertebral body.
2. This unstable injury, caused by hyperextension, is associated with ligamentous tears and possible spinal cord compression.

CHAPTER 10

TEST CASES 9, 10, AND 11

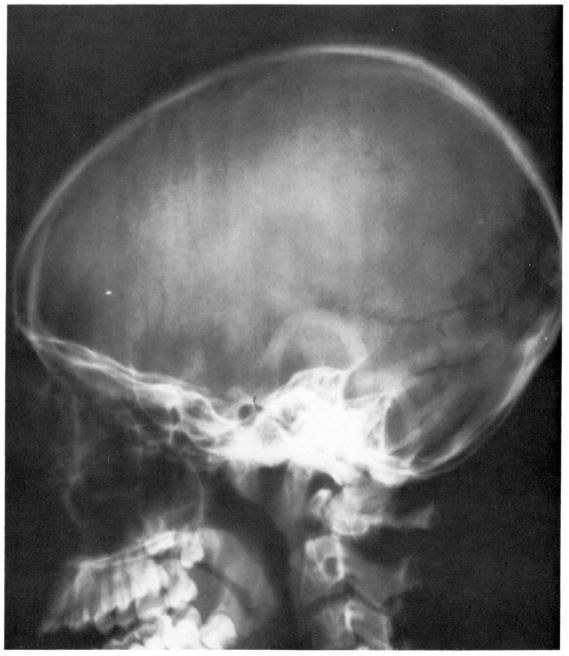

FIGURE 43
Test Case 9

TEST CASE 9

WHAT IS YOUR DIAGNOSIS?

1. Which anatomic structure or structures are involved? _____

_____

_____

2. Are the involved structures displaced or nondisplaced? _____

_____

_____

3. Is this a stable or an unstable injury? _____

_____

_____

4. What is the common eponym or diagnostic term for the type of injury seen on the radiograph? _____

_____

_____

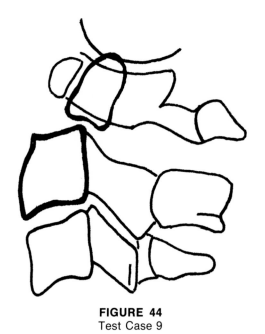

FIGURE 44
Test Case 9

ANSWERS:

1. Which anatomic structure or structures are involved? *Fracture of the base of the dens*

2. Are the involved structures displaced or nondisplaced? *Posterior displacement of C-1 and the dens on C-2*

3. Is this a stable or an unstable injury? *Unstable*

4. What is the common eponym or diagnostic term for the type of injury seen on the radiograph? *Atlanto-axial subluxation, with fracture of the dens or odontoid process*

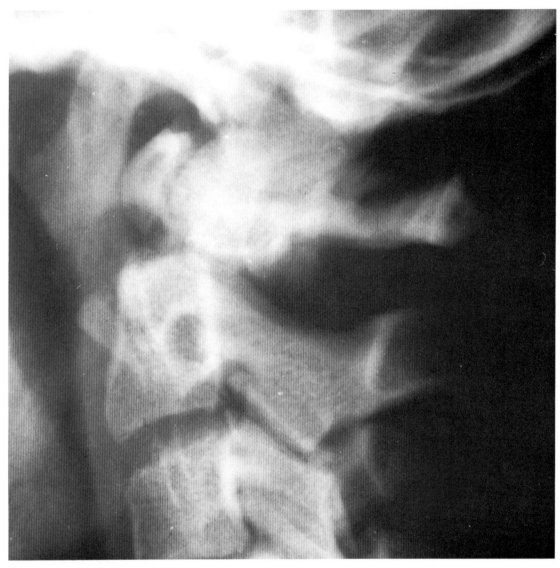

FIGURE 45
Test Case 10

TEST CASE 10

WHAT IS YOUR DIAGNOSIS?

1. Which anatomic structure or structures are involved? _____

_____

_____

2. Are the involved structures displaced or nondisplaced? _____

_____

_____

3. Is this a stable or an unstable injury? _____

_____

_____

4. What is the common eponym or diagnostic term for the type of injury seen on the radiograph? _____

_____

_____

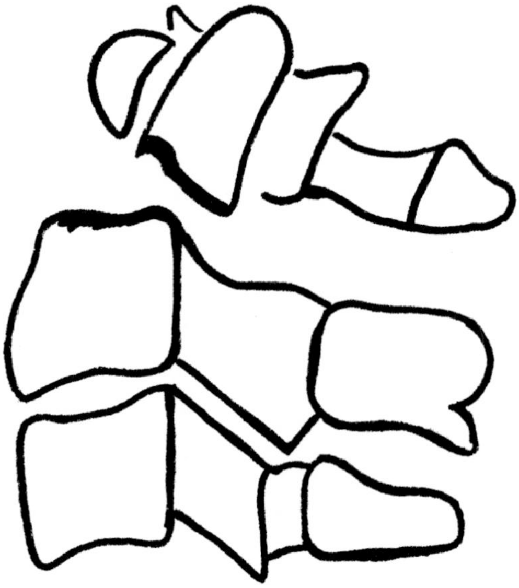

FIGURE 46
Test Case 10

TEST CASE 10

ANSWERS:

1. Which anatomic structure or structures are involved? *Fracture of the dens*

2. Are the involved structures displaced or nondisplaced? *Posterior displacement of the C-1 and the dens on C-2*

3. Is this a stable or an unstable injury? *Unstable*

4. What is the common eponym or diagnostic term for the type of injury seen on the radiograph? *Fracture of the dens with posterior atlanto-axial subluxation*

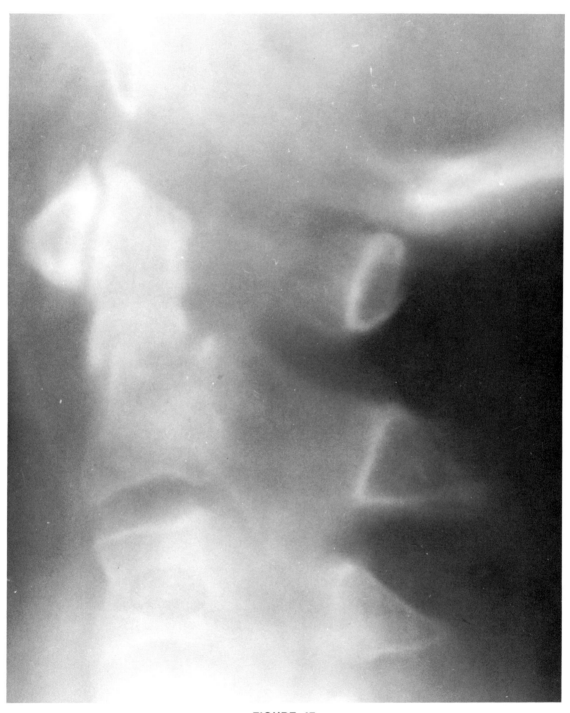

FIGURE 47
Test Case 11

TEST CASE 11

WHAT IS YOUR DIAGNOSIS?

1. Which anatomic structure or structures are involved? _____

   _____

   _____

2. Are the involved structures displaced or nondisplaced? _____

   _____

   _____

3. Is this a stable or an unstable injury? _____

   _____

   _____

4. What is the common eponym or diagnostic term for the type of injury seen on the radiograph? _____

   _____

   _____

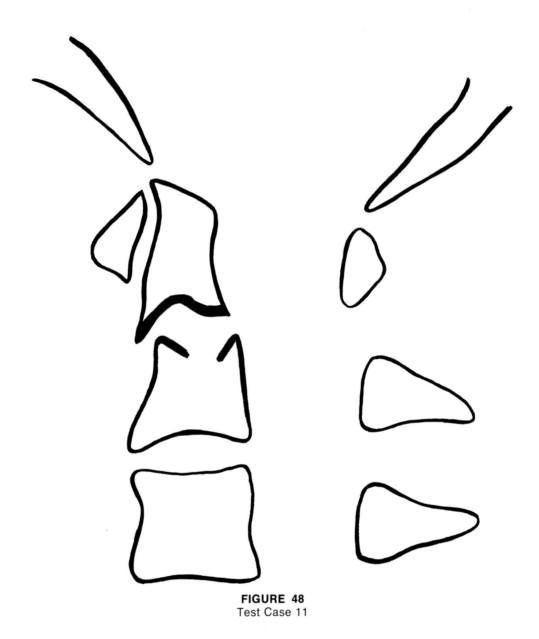

FIGURE 48
Test Case 11

TEST CASE 11

ANSWERS:

1. Which anatomic structure or structures are involved? *Fracture of the dens*

2. Are the involved structures displaced or nondisplaced? *Anterior subluxation of the dens and C-1 on C-2*

3. Is this a stable or an unstable injury? *Unstable*

4. What is the common eponym or diagnostic term for the type of injury seen on the radiograph? *Fracture of the dens, with anterior atlanto-axial subluxation*

Fracture of the Dens

Fractures of the dens can occur with either forced hyperflexion or forced hyperextension of the head on the neck. In hyperflexion injuries, the dens is displaced anteriorly and there is forward subluxation of C-1 on C-2 (Fig. 49). Hyperextension injuries cause the dens to be displaced posteriorly, and there is posterior subluxation of C-1 on C-2 (Fig. 50).

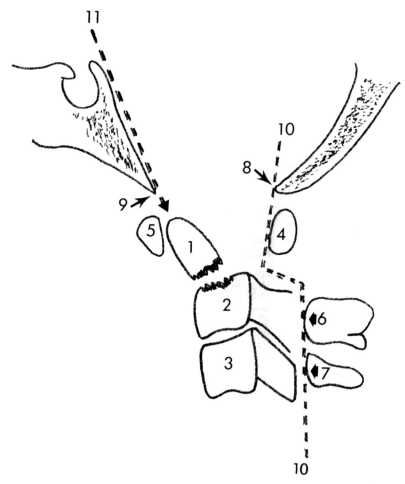

FIGURE 49

Fracture of the dens with anterior subluxation of C-1 on C-2.
1. Dens
2. Body of C-2
3. Body of C-3
4. Posterior arch of C-1
5. Anterior arch of C-1
6. Base of the spinous process of C-2
7. Base of the spinous process of C-3
8. Posterior rim of the foramen magnum
9. Anterior rim of the foramen magnum
10. Contour line 3, the spinolaminal line
11. Line drawn down the clivus adjacent to the anterior rim of the foramen magnum, pointing to the tip of the dens

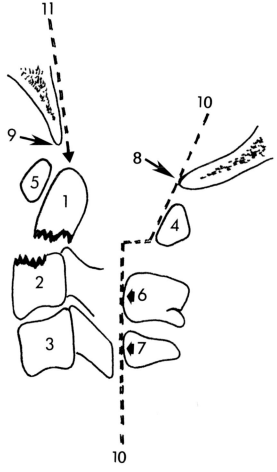

FIGURE 50

Fracture of the dens with posterior subluxation of C-1 on C-2.
1. Dens
2. Vertebral body of C-2
3. Vertebral body of C-3
4. Posterior arch of C-1
5. Anterior arch of C-1
6. Base of the spinous process of C-2
7. Base of the spinous process of C-3
8. Posterior rim of the foramen magnum
9. Anterior rim of the foramen magnum
10. Contour line 3, the spinolaminal line
11. Line drawn down the clivus adjacent to the anterior rim of the foramen magnum, pointing to the dens

Figure 47 demonstrates a fracture through the base of the dens and is included to show the anatomy of the anterior and posterior rims of the foramen magnum and their relationship to the tip of the dens and the posterior arch of C-1. Study this figure closely and notice how the anterior rim of the foramen magnum points to the tip of the dens. Also, examine the posterior rim of the foramen magnum and notice that it points to and forms a smooth contour with the spinolaminal surface of the posterior arch of C-1. These points are in correct alignment, showing that the occipito-atlantal joints are intact.

What is abnormal is the "step-off" configuration in the dotted line drawn adjacent to the spinolaminal surfaces of C-1 and C-2 (Fig. 47 and 49). This "step-off" configuration denotes forward subluxation of C-1 on C-2.

Posterior displacement of C-1 is associated with a posteriorly displaced dens fracture (Figs. 43, 45, and 50). This is a result of the head and C-1 being posteriorly displaced, pulling the dens back. Where C-1 goes so goes the dens unless there is a rupture of the transverse ligament.

Fractures of the dens can also occur without subluxation of C-1 on C-2. In these injuries, the fracture line involving the dens runs transversely across its base, which is that portion of the dens which joins it to the cancellous bone of the body of C-2 (Fig. 51). The fracture line involving the base of the dens frequently extends downward to involve the body of the axis.

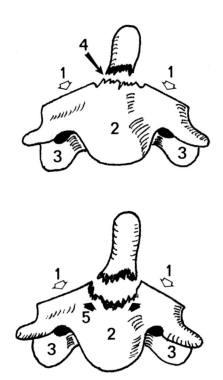

FIGURE 51

Anteroposterior views of the C-2 vertebra, showing site of fractures of the dens.
1. Superior articular facets of C-2
2. Vertebral body of C-2
3. Inferior articular facets of C-2
4. Transverse fracture through the base of the dens
5. Fracture of the base of the dens extending into the cancellous bone of the body of C-2

Fractures of the dens without displacement or subluxation of C-1 on C-2 can be most difficult to recognize. Laminagraphy or polytomography of the dens in the anteroposterior and lateral projections may be helpful in detecting these fractures. This technique can be used whenever the patient has a history suggestive of a fracture of the dens and the diagnosis is uncertain from the routine views of the cervical spine. A mid-sagittal plane laminagram of the occipito-atlanto-axial joint is shown in Figure 47.

Suppose that you see a fracture of the dens with an associated increase in the space between the anterior arch of the atlas and the dens; what would be your diagnosis? Correct, if you said fracture of the dens and a rupture of the transverse ligament, too. A rare combination, but it certainly might happen.

All lateral radiographic views of the skull include a lateral view of the dens and the occipito-atlanto-axial joints. Failure to appreciate this fact can get you into trouble when evaluating the skull series of an acutely injured patient. To emphasize this point, several lateral skull radiographs demonstrating cervical spine trauma have been included in this monograph.

Summary of the Radiographic Findings in Dens Fractures

1. The fracture line occurs at the base of the dens and may extend into the body of C-2.
2. Anterior or posterior displacement of the dens and C-1 may occur.
3. A zigzag or "step-off" configuration of contour lines drawn adjacent to the bases of the spinous processes of C-1 and C-2 indicates that C-1 has subluxed either anteriorly or posteriorly on C-2.

CHAPTER 11
TEST CASE 12

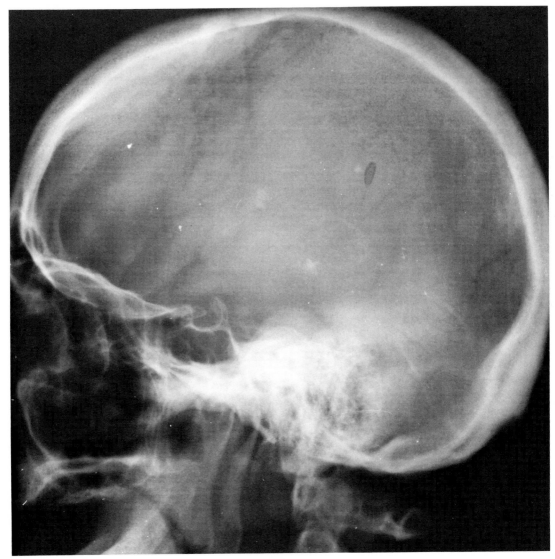

FIGURE 52
Test Case 12

TEST CASE 12

WHAT IS YOUR DIAGNOSIS?

1. Which anatomic structure or structures are involved? _____

_____

_____

2. Are the involved structures displaced or nondisplaced? _____

_____

_____

3. Is this a stable or an unstable injury? _____

_____

_____

4. What is the common eponym or diagnostic term for the type of injury
   seen on the radiograph? _____

_____

_____

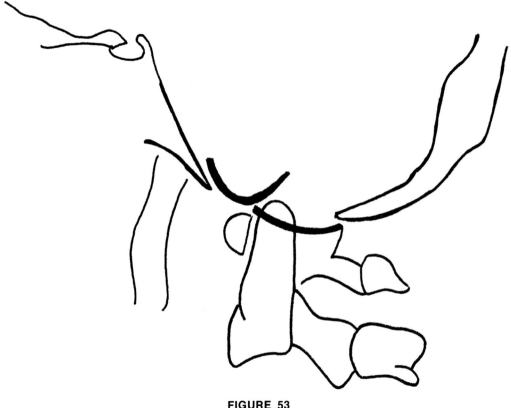

FIGURE 53
Test Case 12

ANSWERS:

1. Which anatomic structure or structures are involved? *There is no fracture. Rather, there is a total dislocation of the head on the neck occurring through the occipito-atlantal joints.*

2. Are the involved structures displaced or nondisplaced? *Of course, the occipital condyles are anteriorly displaced.*

3. Is this a stable or an unstable injury? *Unstable.*

4. What is the common eponym or diagnostic term for the type of injury seen on the radiograph? *Occipito-atlantal dislocation.*

The occipital condyles lie anterior to the superior articular facets of C-1. A clue to the diagnosis of occipito-atlantal dislocation is an abnormally wide space between the mandibular rami and the dens (Fig. 55).

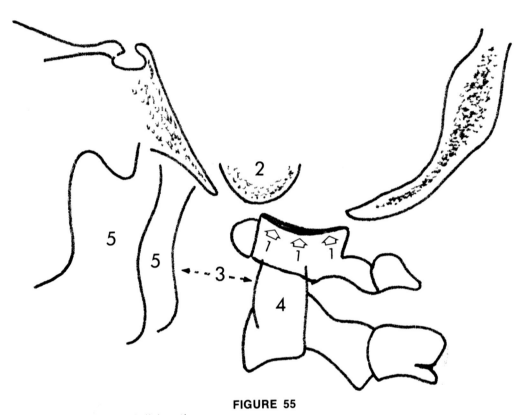

FIGURE 55

Occipito-atlantal dislocation.
1. Superior articular facet of C-1
2. Occipital condyle
3. A dotted line showing an increase in the space between the posterior margin of the rami of the mandible and the anterior margin of the dens
4. Body of C-2
5. Rami of the mandible

Summary of the Radiographic Findings in Occipito-Atlantal Dislocations

1. There is displacement of the anterior rim of the foramen magnum in front of the dens.
2. There is displacement of the posterior rim of the foramen magnum in front of the posterior arch of C-1.
3. Anterior dislocations of the occipital condyles occur with respect to the superior articular facets of C-1.

CHAPTER 12

TEST CASE 13

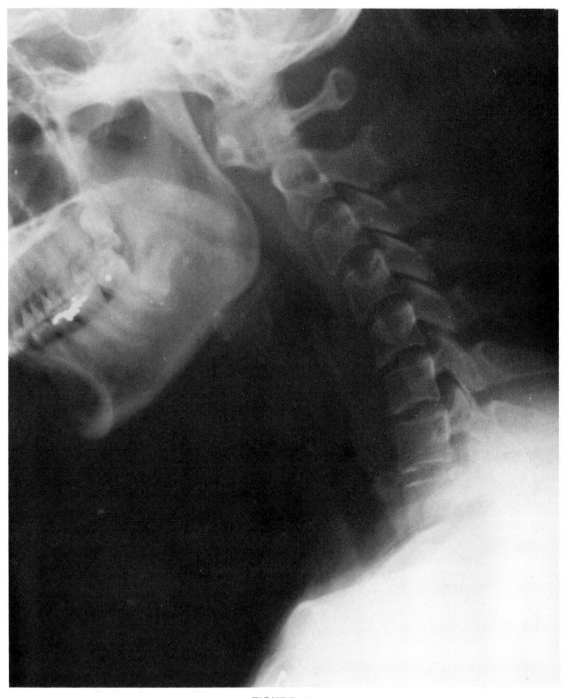

FIGURE 56
Test Case 13

TEST CASE 13

WHAT IS YOUR DIAGNOSIS?

1. Which anatomic structure or structures are involved? _____

   _____

   _____

2. Are the involved structures displaced or nondisplaced? _____

   _____

   _____

3. Is this a stable or an unstable injury? _____

   _____

   _____

4. What is the common eponym or diagnostic term for the type of injury
   seen on the radiograph? _____

   _____

   _____

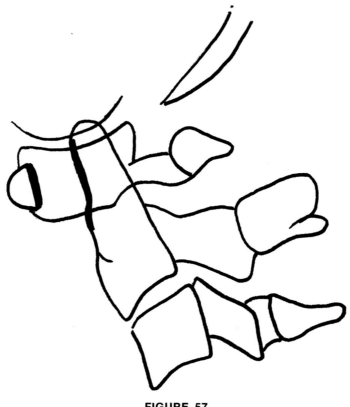

FIGURE 57
Test Case 13

TEST CASE 13

ANSWERS:

1. Which anatomic structure or structures are involved? *There is a rupture of the transverse ligament of C-1. No fractures are present.*

2. Are the involved structures displaced or nondisplaced? *C-1 is displaced anteriorly with respect to the odontoid process of C-2.*

3. Is this a stable or an unstable injury? *Unstable*

4. What is the common eponym or diagnostic term for the type of injury seen on the radiograph? *Atlanto-axial subluxation*

Atlanto-Axial Subluxation

Atlanto-axial subluxation is partial disruption of the normal contact between the articular surfaces of C-1 and C-2. Subluxation of C-1 on C-2 can be the result of a fracture of the dens or a rupture of the transverse ligament. In the normal individual, the transverse ligament is stronger than the odontoid process, so the odontoid process will fracture before the transverse ligament ruptures. However, if the transverse ligament is weakened by some disease process, such as rheumatoid arthritis or inflammation in the nasopharyngeal region, it will rupture before the dens fractures. Since the transverse ligament forms a part of the synovial joint about the odontoid process, it is easy to see how it could be weakened in rheumatoid arthritis. Tonsillitis, pharyngitis, and cervical adenitis also can cause the transverse ligament to become weak and predisposed to rupture. Presumably, this effect is due to the lymphatic communication between retropharyngeal lymph nodes and their proximity to the synovial joint space about the transverse ligament. Whatever the cause of the weakened transverse ligament, severe flexion of the head on the neck or a severe blow to the back of the head can certainly rupture the abnormal ligament, causing the atlas to sublux anteriorly on the axis.

In Figure 58A the transverse ligament is intact; in Figure 58B it is torn. Notice that when the transverse ligament is intact, the anterior arch of C-1 is fixed firmly against the anterior margin of the odontoid process. With the rupture of the transverse ligament, the anterior arch of the atlas is no longer fixed; instead, it is free to move forward, and the space between it and the odontoid process becomes wider. One of the diagnostic signs of an atlanto-axial subluxation (caused by rupture of a transverse ligament) is, therefore, an increased distance between the anterior arch of C-1 and the anterior surface of the odontoid process. Since the atlas is a ring-shaped structure, the posterior arch of C-1 must move forward when the anterior arch does.

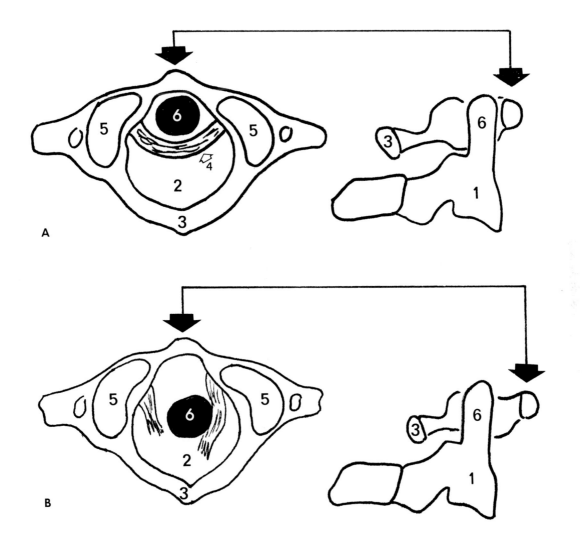

FIGURE 58

Atlanto-axial subluxation. *A*, Intact transverse ligament. *B*, Ruptured transverse ligament.

1. Body of C-2
2. Spinal canal
3. Posterior arch of C-1
4. Transverse ligament
5. Superior articular facets of C-1
6. Odontoid process

A second diagnostic sign of atlanto-axial subluxation is forward displacement of the posterior arch of the atlas. This can be recognized by the "step-off" configuration of the spinolaminal line at C-1 and C-2 (Fig. 59). Also, note in Figure 59 how the spinal cord is compressed against the posterior aspect of the dens by the anteriorly displaced posterior arch of the atlas. It is this "pinch-cock" compression of the spinal cord between the dens and the posterior arch of C-1 that makes this injury unstable and deleterious to the patient.

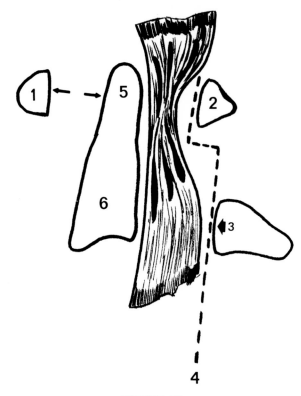

FIGURE 59
Compression of the spinal cord due to atlanto-axial subluxation.
1. Anterior arch of C-1
2. Posterior arch of C-1
3. Base of the spinous process of C-2
4. Line drawn adjacent to the base of the tubercle (spinous process) of C-1 and base of the spinous process of C-2, showing a "step-off" configuration
5. Dens
6. Body of C-2

Summary of the Radiographic Findings in Atlanto-Axial Subluxation

1. There is an increase in the space between the anterior arch of C-1 and the dens.
2. The space between the posterior arch of C-1 and the dens is narrow.
3. There is a "step-off" configuration in a line drawn adjacent to the bases of the spinous processes of C-1 and C-2.

CHAPTER 13

TEST CASES 14 AND 15

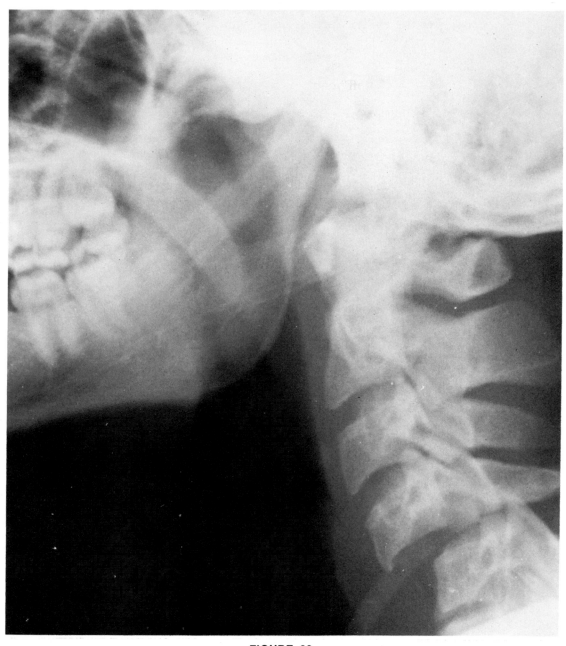

FIGURE 60
Test Case 14

TEST CASE 14

WHAT IS YOUR DIAGNOSIS?

1. Which anatomic structure or structures are involved? _____

_____

_____

2. Are the involved structures displaced or nondisplaced? _____

_____

_____

3. Is this a stable or an unstable injury? _____

_____

_____

4. What is the common eponym or diagnostic term for the type of injury seen on the radiograph? _____

_____

_____

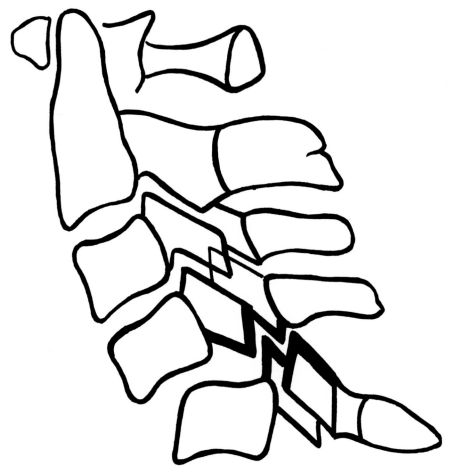

FIGURE 61
Test Case 14

TEST CASE 14

ANSWERS:

1. Which anatomic structure or structures are involved? *There are no fractures. The C-4 and C-5 vertebral bodies are involved.*

2. Are the involved structures displaced or nondisplaced? *Both inferior articular processes of C-4 are dislocated anterior to both superior articular processes of C-5.*

3. Is this a stable or an unstable injury? *Unstable*

4. What is the common eponym or diagnostic term for the type of injury seen on the radiograph? *Bilateral "locked" facets*

Interlocking Articular Facets

Extreme flexion of the head and neck on the body is necessary to dislocate the articular facets. The separation of vertebral segments tears the supporting ligaments, allowing the articular facets to dislocate and interlock.

Interlocking of the articular facets begins with the movement of the inferior articular facets of one vertebra forward over the superior articular facets of the underlying vertebra. The inferior facets move forward and up the slope formed by the superior facets. This causes the laminae and spinous processes of the vertebrae to spread apart and the vertebral bodies to sublux. Figure 62A shows that the inferior facets of the shaded vertebra have moved forward and upward on the superior facets of the vertebra below it. The tips of the inferior articular processes of the shaded vertebra are "perched" on the tips of the superior articular processes of the vertebra below it. The spinous processes and laminae are spread apart, disrupting the ligamenta flava and the supraspinous and interspinous cervical ligaments (Fig. 63A). The apophyseal joints

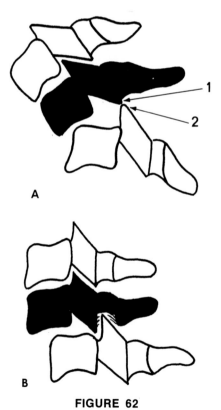

FIGURE 62

Mechanism of interlocking articular facets. *A*, Tips of the inferior articular facets (1) of one vertebra (shaded) "perched" on the tips of the superior facets (2) of the vertebra below it. *B*, Tips of the inferior articular facets of one vertebra (shaded) locked in front of the tips of the superior facets of the vertebra below it.

are totally disrupted, as are the capsular ligaments. The anterior and posterior longitudinal ligaments may also be damaged (Fig. 63B). Should the tips of the inferior facets of the shaded vertebra continue to move forward, they would slide over and in front of the peaks formed by the tips of the superior facets of the vertebra below, causing complete dislocation and locking (Fig. 62B). Since the inferior facets of the shaded vertebra have moved forward on the superior facets of the vertebra below, the entire shaded vertebra must be displaced anteriorly. A "step-off" configuration in the contour lines along the anterior and posterior surfaces of the involved vertebral bodies occurs (Fig. 64). The base of the

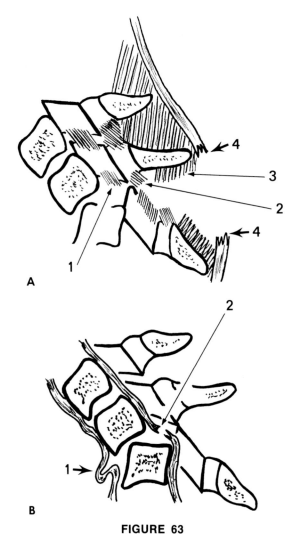

FIGURE 63

Ligamentous injuries associated with interlocking articular facets.

A:

    1. Rupture of the capsular ligaments
    2. Rupture of the ligamenta flava
    3. Rupture of the interspinous ligament
    4. Rupture of the supraspinous ligament

B:

    1. Detached anterior longitudinal ligament
    2. Ruptured posterior longitudinal ligament

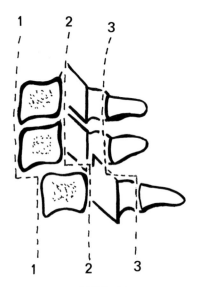

FIGURE 64

Disruption of the contour lines of the cervical spine due to interlocking of the articular facets.

1. "Step-off" configuration of the line drawn along the anterior surface of the vertebral bodies
2. "Step-off" configuration of the line drawn along the posterior surfaces of the vertebral bodies
3. "Step-off" configuration of the spinolaminal line

spinous process of the shaded vertebra is also displaced forward on the base of the spinous process of the vertebra below. This causes narrowing of the anteroposterior diameter of the spinal canal and a "step-off" configuration of the spinolaminal line (Figs. 64 and 65).

When the mechanism of injury is flexion and rotation, a unilateral dislocation and unilateral locked facet may occur. In this situation, the radiographic findings may be more subtle. There is usually less forward displacement of the involved vertebral body. The key to recognition is that while the vertebrae below are in the true lateral projection, the vertebrae above are seen obliquely (Fig. 66). This results in a "bowtie" or "bat-wing" appearance of the articular pillars of the dislocated vertebra (Figs. 66 and 67).

Fractures of the vertebral bodies, articular processes, laminae, and spinous processes may be associated with injuries that cause dislocation of the articular facets.

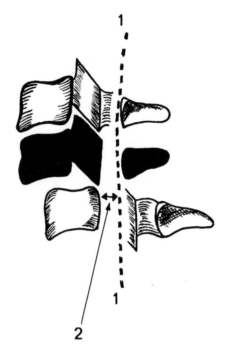

FIGURE 65

Narrowing of the spinal canal with interlocking of the articular facets.
1. Line drawn adjacent to the base of the spinous process of the anteriorly displaced and locked black vertebral body
2. Arrows show the anteroposterior diameter of the narrowed spinal canal. The measurement of the anteroposterior diameter of the spinal canal is taken at its narrowest point. With interlocking facets, the measurement is taken from a line drawn adjacent to the base of the spinous process of the dislocated vertebra to the posterior margin of the vertebral body below.

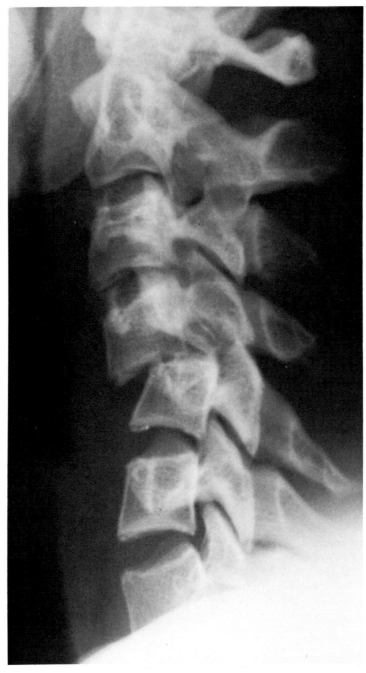

FIGURE 66
Unilateral locked facet

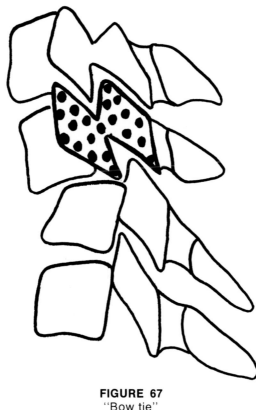

FIGURE 67
"Bow tie"

Summary of the Radiographic Findings with Interlocking of the Articular Facets

1. There is anterior displacement of the affected vertebra.
2. One or both articular processes may be locked.
3. A "step-off" configuration of the contour lines is noted.
4. Ligamentous structures are disrupted.
5. The spinal canal is narrowed.

CHAPTER 14

TEST CASE 16

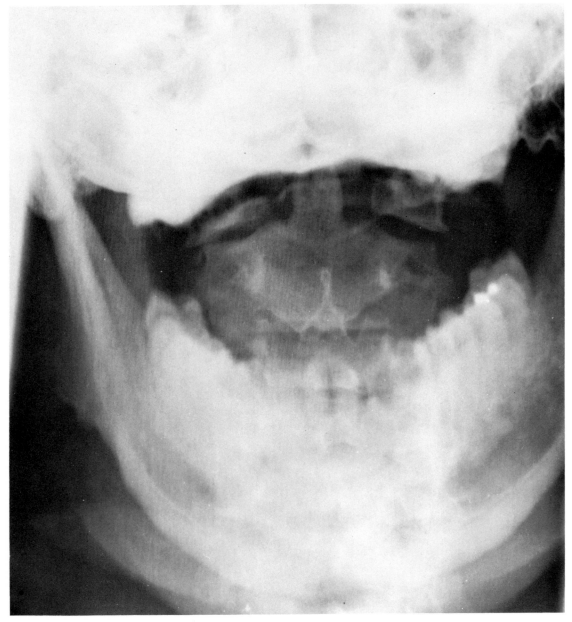

FIGURE 68
Test Case 16

WHAT IS YOUR DIAGNOSIS?

1. Which anatomic structure or structures are involved? _____

_____

_____

2. Are the involved structures displaced or nondisplaced? _____

_____

_____

3. Is this a stable or an unstable injury? _____

_____

_____

4. What is the common eponym or diagnostic term for the type of injury
seen on the radiograph? _____

_____

_____

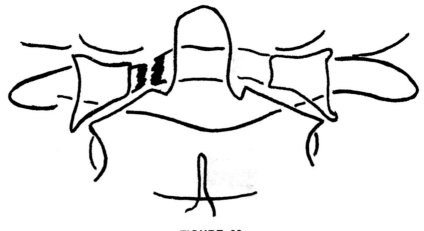

FIGURE 69
Test Case 16

TEST CASE 16

ANSWERS:

1. Which anatomic structure or structures are involved? *There are fractures of the ring of C-1.*

2. Are the involved structures displaced or nondisplaced? *There are bilateral lateral displacements of the lateral masses of C-1.*

3. Is this a stable or an unstable injury? *Unstable*

4. What is the common eponym or diagnostic term for the type of injury seen on the radiograph? *Jefferson fracture*

Jefferson Fracture

Sir Geoffrey Jefferson first called attention to this fracture involving the C-1 vertebra when he presented the mechanism of injury in 1920. Since that time, the fracture has come to bear his name. What is it and how do you get it? Try diving off a raft at low tide and see what happens. Wow! I bet that "smarts." (One of the authors did and she says that it does indeed!)

The Jefferson fracture is a compression or bursting fracture of C-1. It is produced by a direct blow to the vertex of the head. This causes the occipital condyles to compress the lateral masses of C-1 against the superior articular facets of C-2. As you recall, C-1 is merely a ring of bone, with its superior and inferior articular facets obliquely oriented so that the lateral masses are wedge-shaped when seen from the front (Fig. 70).

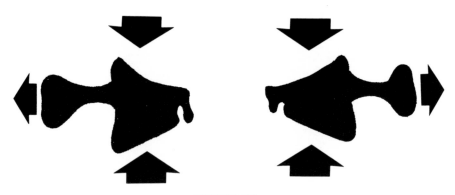

FIGURE 70
Mechanism of injury of Jefferson fracture

Any compression force on these wedge-shaped lateral masses of C-1 tends to spread them apart (Fig. 70). If the force is great enough, the ring of bone forming the C-1 vertebra will burst. The bursting usually occur in four places—two anteriorly and two posteriorly (Fig. 71). The lateral displacement of the lateral masses enlarges the transverse diameter of the spinal canal. If the transverse ligament remains intact, no neurologic deficit will occur. If the transverse ligament is ruptured by the lateral displacement of the lateral masses, the C-1 vertebra can slip forward on the C-2 vertebra and compress the spinal cord, causing neurologic deficit.

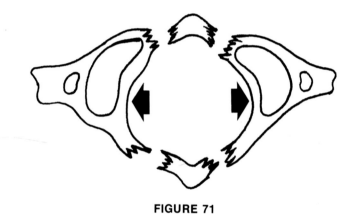

FIGURE 71
Jefferson fracture

When the transverse ligament remains intact and there is no forward displacement of C-1 on C-2, the plain lateral radiograph of the cervical spine will appear normal. It is for this reason that the anteroposterior odontoid view is so important in the diagnosis of this fracture. Normally on the anteroposterior view the lateral margins of the articular pillars of C-2 line up with the lateral margins of the lateral masses of C-1 (Fig. 72A). If the ring of C-1 is disrupted, there is bilateral lateral displacement of the lateral masses of C-1 with respect to the pillars of C-2.

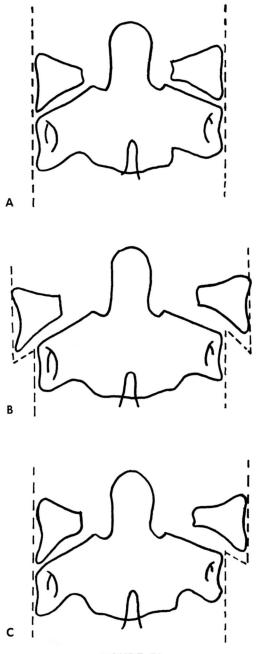

FIGURE 72
Relationship of C-1 to C-2

Now there will be a "step-off" or zigzag configuration in a line drawn adjacent to these structures (Fig. 72B). If both lines zigzag laterally, the patient must have a Jefferson fracture. Now, let's consider Figure 73. Does this patient have a Jefferson fracture? In this case, one line zigzags medially while the other line zigzags laterally. The patient does not have a Jefferson fracture at all; rather, the radiographic findings are due to rotation of the head.

What if the line on one side is straight while the other line zigzags laterally? Does that patient have a Jefferson fracture (Fig. 72C)? Think about it. The answer is yes. This type of configuration can only exist if the ring of C-1 is broken.

Sometimes you will actually be able to see the fractures of the ring of C-1 on the plain anteroposterior odontoid view, but you do not have to identify fracture lines to make the diagnosis of a Jefferson fracture.

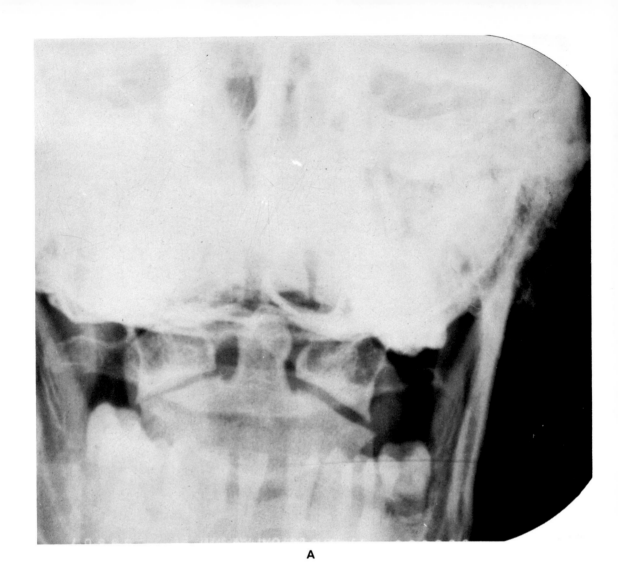

A

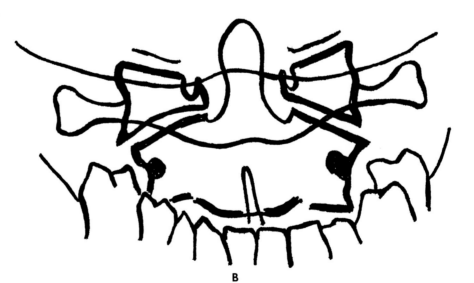

B

FIGURE 73

Summary of the Radiographic Findings in Jefferson Fracture

1. Bilateral lateral displacement of the lateral masses of C-1 with respect to the articular pillars of C-2.
2. Unilateral lateral displacement of a lateral mass of C-1 if there is no compensatory medial movement of the opposite lateral mass.
3. The fracture lines may or may not be directly visualized on routine radiographs.

CHAPTER 15

TEST CASES 17, 18, 19, AND 20

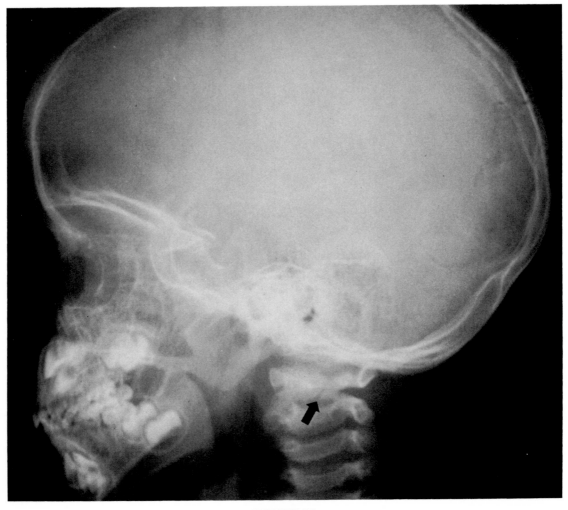

FIGURE 74
Test Case 17

TEST CASE 17

WHAT IS YOUR DIAGNOSIS?

1. Which anatomic structure or structures are involved? _____

   _____

   _____

2. Are the involved structures displaced or nondisplaced? _____

   _____

   _____

3. Is this a stable or an unstable injury? _____

   _____

   _____

4. What is the common eponym or diagnostic term for the type of injury seen on the radiograph? _____

   _____

   _____

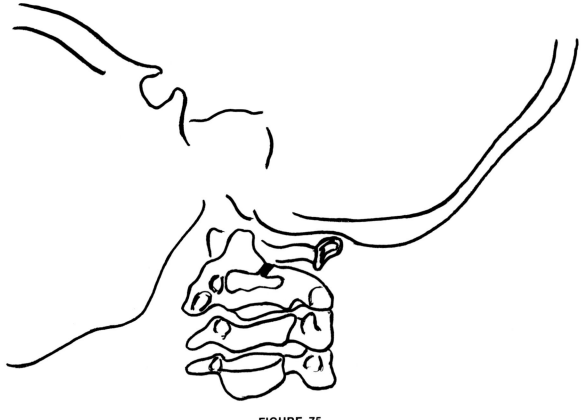

FIGURE 75
Test Case 17

TEST CASE 17

ANSWERS:

1. Which anatomic structure or structures are involved? *There is no fracture. The lucent shadow at the end of the arrow is a cleft in the neural arch of the atlas, a normal variant. This cleft usually ossifies by the age of seven.*

2. Are the involved structures displaced or nondisplaced? *Not relevant*

3. Is this a stable or an unstable injury? *Not relevant*

4. What is the common eponym or diagnostic term for the type of injury seen on the radiograph? *Not relevant*

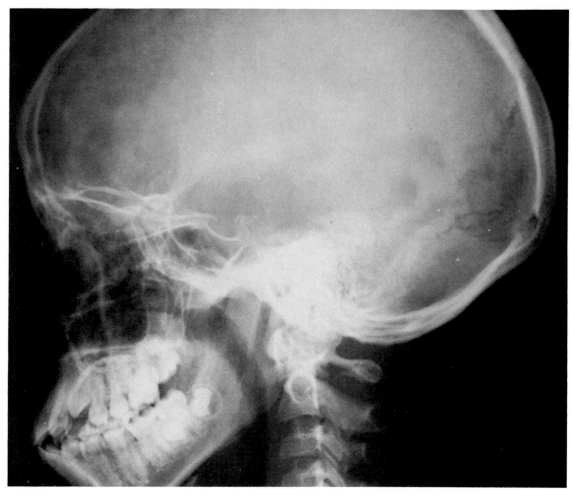

FIGURE 76
Test Case 18

TEST CASE 18

WHAT IS YOUR DIAGNOSIS?

1. Which anatomic structure or structures are involved?_____

_____

_____

2. Are the involved structures displaced or nondisplaced? _____

_____

_____

3. Is this a stable or an unstable injury? _____

_____

_____

4. What is the common eponym or diagnostic term for the type of injury seen on the radiograph? _____

_____

_____

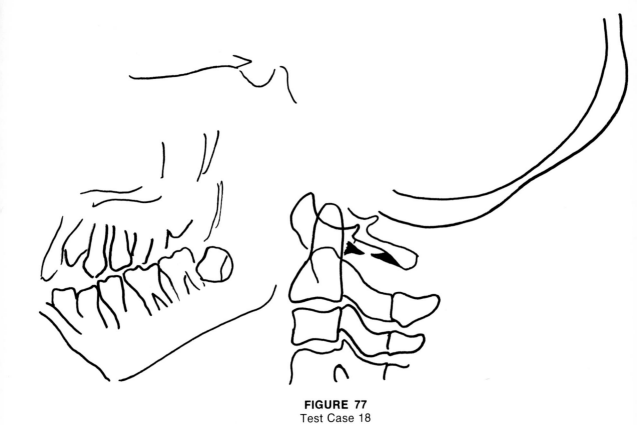

FIGURE 77
Test Case 18

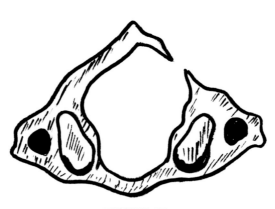

FIGURE 78
Incomplete ossification of C-1

TEST CASE 18

ANSWERS:

1. Which anatomic structure or structures are involved? *There is unilateral absence of a portion of the neural arch of C-1, another normal variant.*

2. Are the involved structures displaced or nondisplaced? *Not relevant*

3. Is this a stable or an unstable injury? *Not relevant*

4. What is the common eponym or diagnostic term for the type of injury seen on the radiograph? *Not relevant*

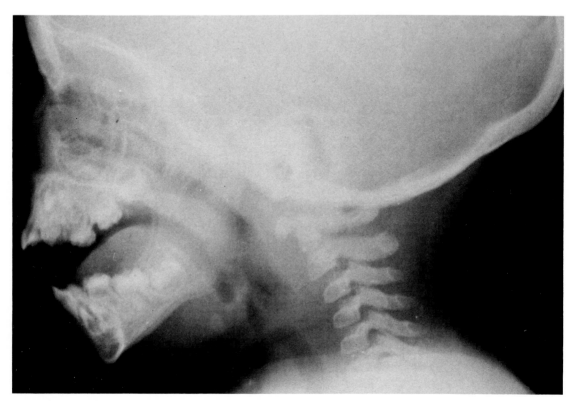

FIGURE 79
Test Case 19

TEST CASE 19

WHAT IS YOUR DIAGNOSIS?

1. Which anatomic structure or structures are involved? _____

_____

_____

2. Are the involved structures displaced or nondisplaced? _____

_____

_____

3. Is this a stable or an unstable injury? _____

_____

_____

4. What is the common eponym or diagnostic term for the type of injury
seen on the radiograph? _____

_____

_____

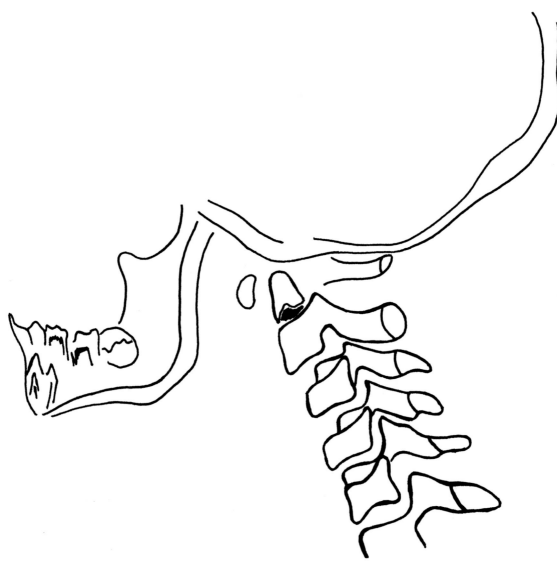

FIGURE 80
Test Case 19

ANSWERS:

1. Which anatomic structure or structures are involved? *The second cervical vertebra ossifies from a number of centers. The lucent line at the junction of the dens with the body of C-2 is a cartilaginous disc, or synchondrosis, which will disappear between the ages of three and seven years. This synchondrosis is a normal finding at the site of fusion of the body of C-2 with the dens and is not a fracture.*

2. Are the involved structures displaced or nondisplaced? *Not relevant*

3. Is this a stable or an unstable injury? *Not relevant*

4. What is the common eponym or diagnostic term for the type of injury seen on the radiograph? *Not relevant*

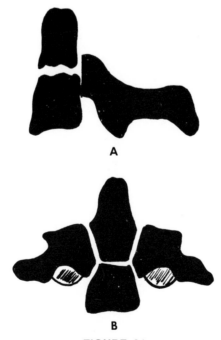

A

B

FIGURE 81

The site of fusion of the dens with the body of C-2 is an area where the uninitiated commonly suspect a fracture.

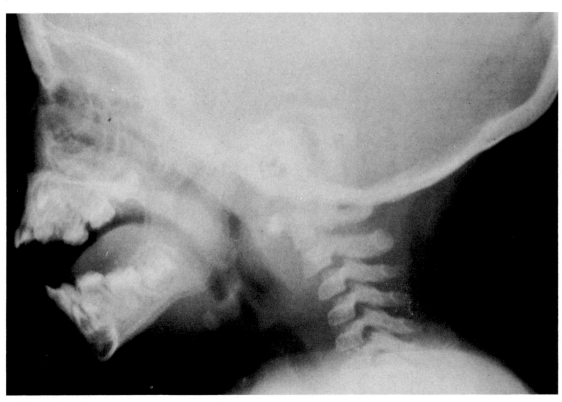

FIGURE 82
Test Case 20

WHAT IS YOUR DIAGNOSIS?

1. Which anatomic structure or structures are involved? _____

_____

_____

2. Are the involved structures displaced or nondisplaced? _____

_____

_____

3. Is this a stable or an unstable injury? _____

_____

_____

4. What is the common eponym or diagnostic term for the type of injury seen on the radiograph? _____

_____

_____

(Look familiar?)

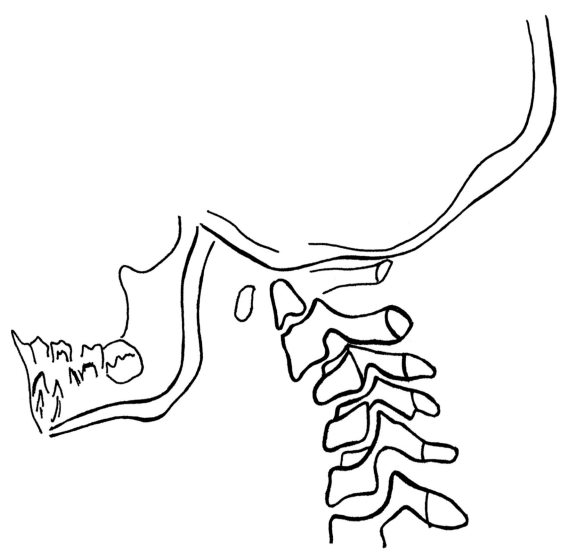

FIGURE 83
Test Case 20

TEST CASE 20

ANSWERS:

1. Which anatomic structure or structures are involved? *Note that C-2 is "subluxed" anteriorly on C-3 (i.e., the first and second contour lines are abnormal). This is a normal physiologic finding in most children. The spinolaminal line is normal. In a hangman's fracture, C-2 would be displaced anteriorly on C-3 and the spinolaminal line projected between C-1 and C-3 would show the posterior arch and spinous process of C-2 displaced posteriorly.*

2. Are the involved structures displaced or nondisplaced? *Not relevant*

3. Is this a stable or an unstable injury? *Not relevant*

4. What is the common eponym or diagnostic term for the type of injury seen on the radiograph? *Not relevant*

   (As you probably noted, this radiograph is the same as Test Case 19, but we wanted to make the above point.)

   The test cases in this chapter were included to emphasize the fact that normal variants may simulate fractures. We have shown you only a few of the many variants.

CHAPTER 16

TEST CASE 21

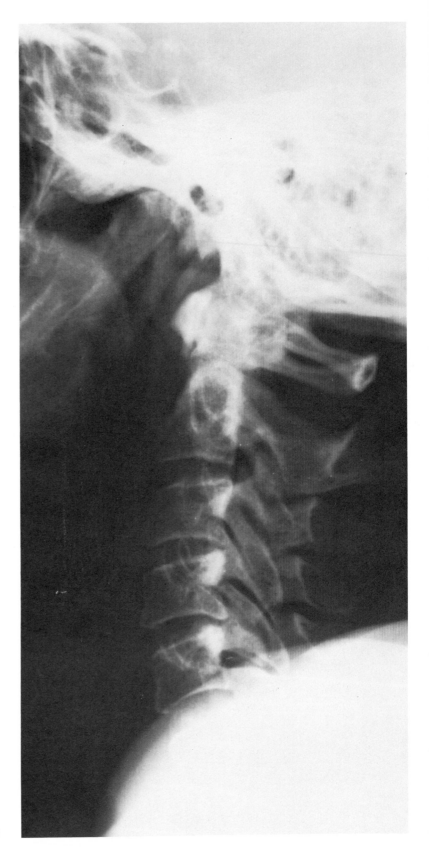

FIGURE 84
Test Case 21

TEST CASE 21

WHAT IS YOUR DIAGNOSIS?

1. Which anatomic structure or structures are involved? _____

   _____

   _____

2. Are the involved structures displaced or nondisplaced? _____

   _____

   _____

3. Is this a stable or an unstable injury? _____

   _____

   _____

4. What is the common eponym or diagnostic term for the type of injury
   seen on the radiograph? _____

   _____

   _____

Surprise! There's no answer sheet.

If you didn't order a repeat lateral view on this poor soul, both you and the patient are in trouble! Figures 85, 86, and 87 will tell you why!

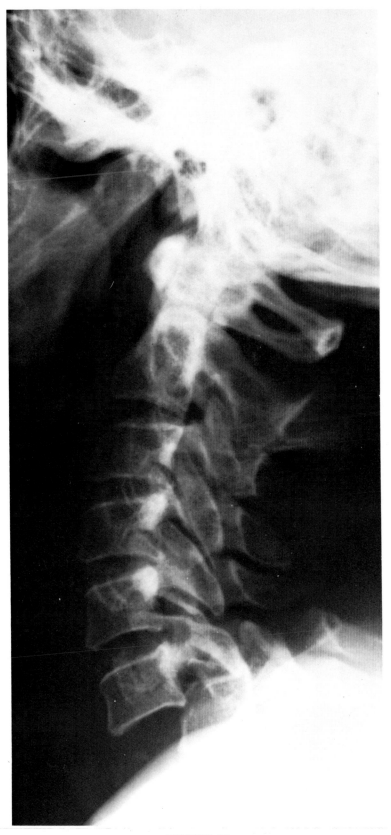

FIGURE 85
Test Case 21

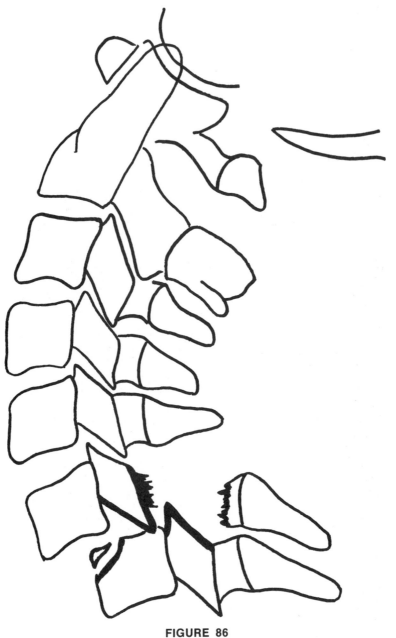

FIGURE 86
Test Case 21

TEST CASE 21

ANSWERS:

1. Which anatomic structure or structures are involved? *The C-6 and C-7 vertebral bodies are involved. There is a fracture of the laminae of C-6 and an anterior compression fracture of C-7.*

2. Are the involved structures displaced or nondisplaced? *C-6 is anteriorly dislocated on C-7, and there are bilaterally interlocked facets.*

3. Is this a stable or an unstable injury? *Unstable*

4. What is the common eponym or diagnostic term for the type of injury seen on the radiograph? *None*

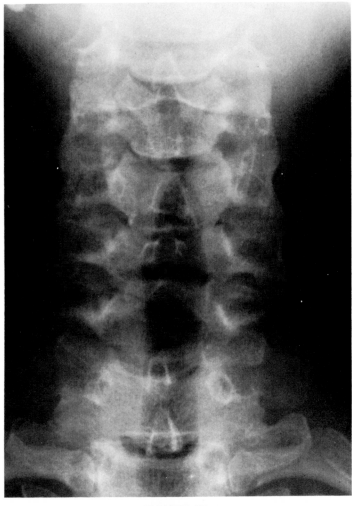

FIGURE 87

Test Case 21. The anteroposterior projection provides a clue to the diagnosis, as there is a separation of the spinous processes.

This test case requires little discussion, as the point has already been made by the radiographs. No lateral view of the cervical spine is acceptable unless seven cervical vertebral bodies are clearly visible. If this cannot be achieved in the standard view, then a so-called "swimmer's" lateral projection should be ordered. For this view, the patient is placed in an oblique position with one arm elevated and the other arm by the side as if he were swimming the crawl. This projection will provide adequate visualization of the cervicothoracic vertebrae, which would otherwise be obscured by the shoulders.

CHAPTER 17

TEST CASES 22 to 30*

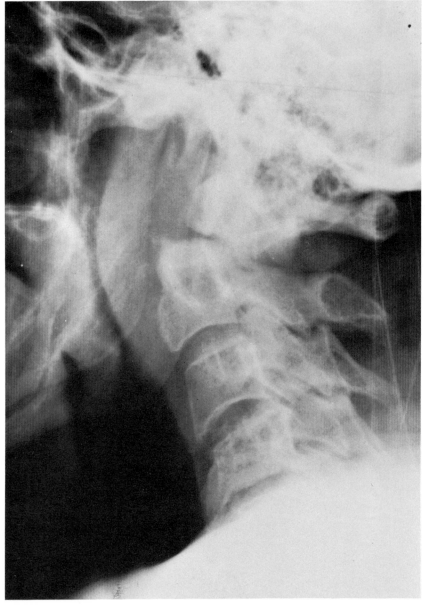

FIGURE 88
Test Case 22

*These test cases are accompanied by multiple choice questions; the answers are listed at the end of the chapter.

TEST CASE 22

Which of the following statements concerning the accompanying radiograph of the cervical spine is/are correct?

A. There is retropharyngeal (prevertebral) soft tissue swelling.
B. There is a fracture of the odontoid.
C. There is an atlanto-axial subluxation.
D. There is a clay shoveler's fracture.
E. There is an occipito-atlantal dislocation.

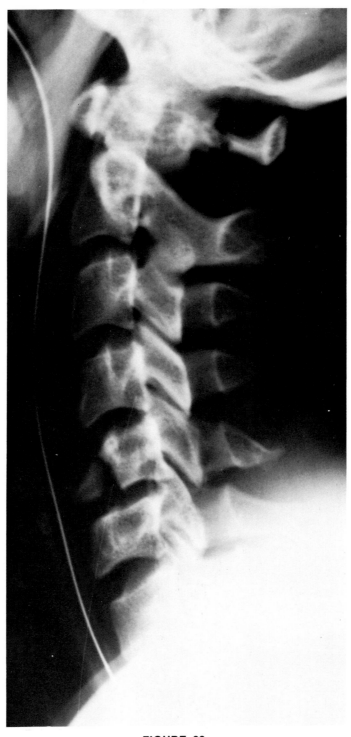

FIGURE 89
Test Case 23

TEST CASE 23

Which of the following statements concerning the accompanying radiograph is/are correct?

A. There is a hangman's fracture.
B. There is a teardrop fracture of C-5.
C. There is a Jefferson fracture.
D. There is a fracture of the posterior neural arch of C-1.
E. There is a subluxation of C-5 on C-6.

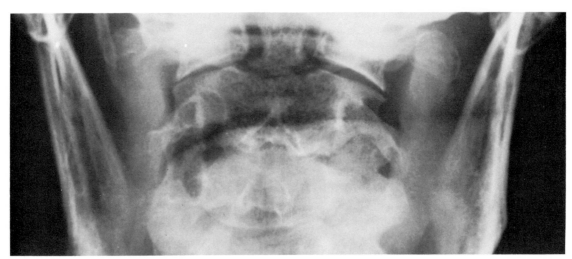

FIGURE 90
Test Case 24

TEST CASE 24

Which of the following statements concerning the accompanying radiograph is/are correct?

A. There is a Jefferson fracture.
B. The radiographic findings are due to rotation of the head.
C. The radiograph illustrates a congenital anomaly.
D. There is a fracture of the odontoid.
E. This is a normal open-mouth view of the odontoid.

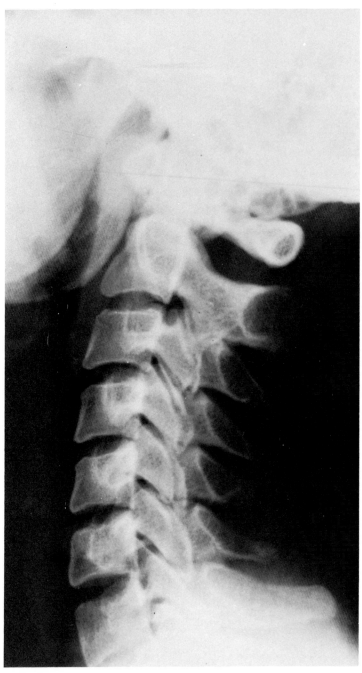

FIGURE 91
Test Case 25

TEST CASE 25

Which of the following statements concerning the accompanying radiograph is/are correct?

A. There is an atlanto-axial subluxation.
B. The radiographic findings are normal.
C. There is a hangman's fracture.
D. There is a clay shoveler's fracture. (Remember the Autobahn?)
E. There is an occipito-atlantal dislocation.

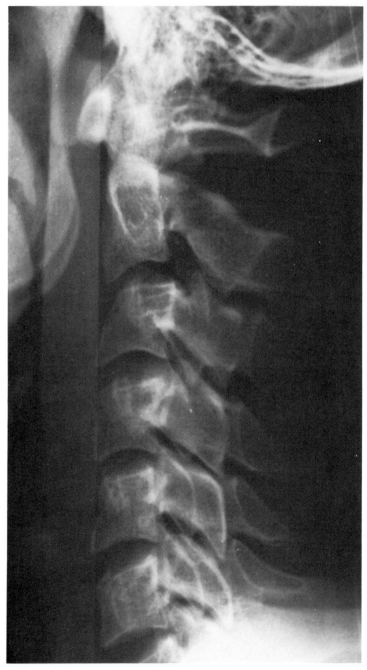

FIGURE 92
Test Case 26

TEST CASE 26

Which of the following statements concerning the accompanying radiograph is/are correct?

A. There is a unilateral locked facet at C-3 on C-4.
B. There is an atlanto-axial subluxation.
C. There is a hangman's fracture.
D. There is a subluxation of C-2 on C-3.
E. There are bilateral pedicle fractures of C-2.

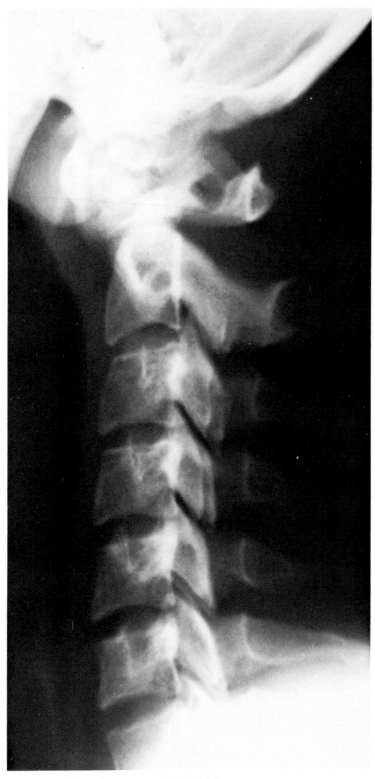

FIGURE 93
Test Case 27

TEST CASE 27

Which of the following statements concerning the accompanying radiograph is/are correct?

A. There is a subluxation of C-1 on C-2.
B. There are bilateral locked facets at C-3 on C-4.
C. There is an odontoid fracture.
D. There is distortion of the prevertebral soft tissues.
E. There is an anterior compression fracture of C-8.

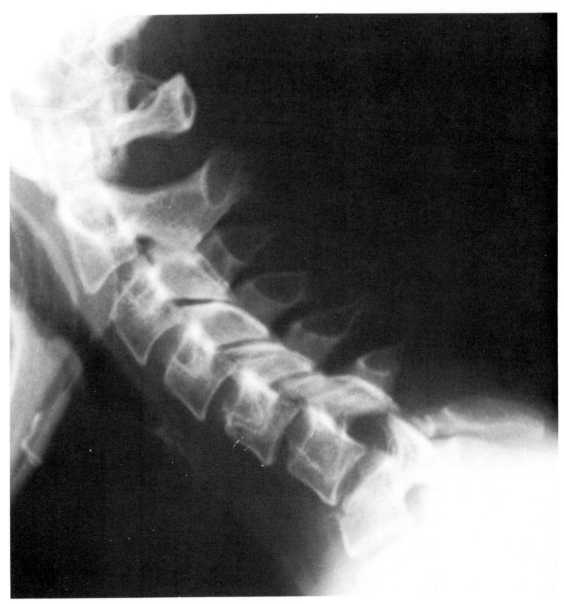

FIGURE 94
Test Case 28

TEST CASE 28

Which of the following statements concerning the accompanying radiograph is/are correct?

A. There is a compression fracture of C-7.
B. There are bilateral interlocked facets.
C. There is a unilateral interlocked facet.
D. There is a clay shoveler's fracture.
E. There is a subluxation of C-6 on C-7.

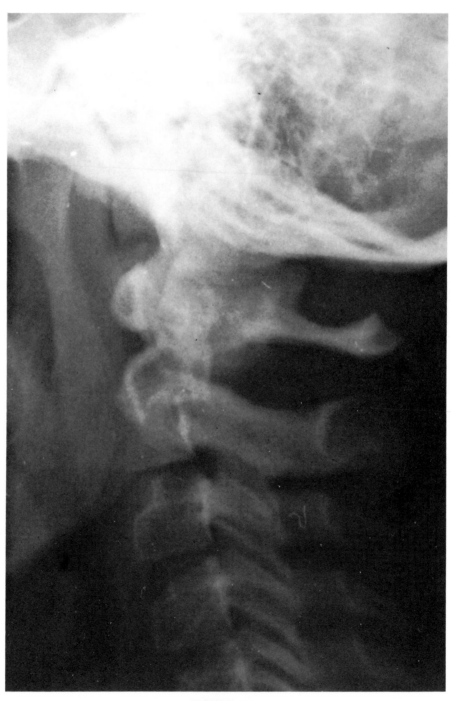

FIGURE 95
Test Case 29

TEST CASE 29

Which of the following statements concerning the accompanying radiograph is/are correct?

A. There is an atlanto-axial subluxation.
B. This is a normal variant.
C. There is a displaced fracture of the odontoid.
D. There is an occipito-atlantal dislocation.
E. There is a hangman's fracture.

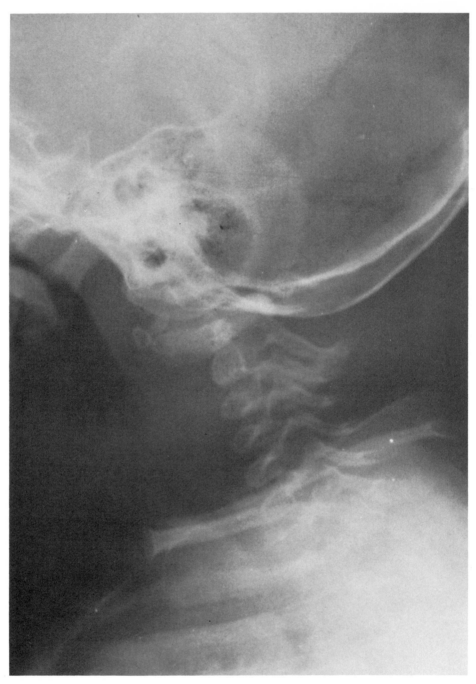

FIGURE 96
Test Case 30

TEST CASE 30

Which of the following statements concerning the accompanying radiograph is/are correct?

A. There is an odontoid fracture.
B. There is an occipito-atlantal dislocation.
C. There are compression fractures of C-4 and C-5.
D. There is a Jefferson fracture.
E. There is an atlanto-axial subluxation.

ANSWERS:

Test Case 22: A, B, and C

Test Case 23: B, D, and E

Test Case 24: D

Test Case 25: B

Test Case 26: C, D, and E

Test Case 27: A, C, and D

Test Case 28: A and E

Test Case 29: C

Test Case 30: E

INDEX